MEDICAL TERMINOLOGY AND THE BODY SYSTEMS

MARY A. COLLIN

MEDICAL TERMINOLOGY AND THE BODY SYSTEMS

Medical Department
Harper & Row, Publishers
Hagerstown, Maryland
New York, Evanston, San Francisco, London

**Library of Congress Cataloging
in Publication Data**

Collin, Mary A. Medical terminology and the
body systems. Bibliography: p. 1. Medicine-
Terminology. 2. Anatomy, Human. I. Title.
[DNLM: 1. Nomenclature. W15 C699m 1974]
R123.C59 — 616'.001'4 — 73-18159. ISBN
0-06-140663-5

CONTENTS

PREFACE

The person who picks up this book to glance through it, or the student who buys the book to learn medical terminology, may wonder: "Who *is* this woman whose book Harper & Row has published? How is she qualified to impart this knowledge with authority?" For this reason, the reader is entitled to some background. A very brief autobiography may be in order.

My mother was a nurse, and through my early years I gained considerable knowledge from her. She was a phenomenal diagnostician. She patiently answered all my questions according to my ability to comprehend. When I began reading well, she gave me all her textbooks to absorb. I wanted to become a doctor, but my father, who was a true Victorian, forbade my attending a school with *men*!

In my teens, I had an uncle who was a doctor; he had five sons, all of whom won scholarships to Washington University in St. Louis, all of whom went on to win Rhodes scholarships, and all of whom became doctors. During the periods of their premed courses, I studied along with them. The six of us conducted our own "seminars" to discuss problems in medical training. They ranged in age from ten years older to two years younger than I — so I had quite a period of study.

At the end of World War II, I went to work for two orthopedic surgeons just returning from war duty, Dr. Maynard M. Conrad and Dr. Curtis M. Hanson. During the five years I worked for them as office nurse and receptionist, they were most helpful in familiarizing me with medical terms, especially orthopedic terms I had not yet learned.

Later, I was employed as a secretary in a large pharmaceutical firm. I was shocked to discover how little the medical secretaries knew of medical terminology. I saw a great need for some type of training, both in spelling the medical terms and in associating these terms with the body system involved. I went to the president of the international division where I worked and asked permission to write a brief textbook and to teach a class of secretaries to understand the terms with which they had to work daily. He was skeptical, but concluded that I could make the attempt, teaching just one class — then we'd "see how that turned out."

That was twelve years ago. Each year, I taught two classes of sixteen weeks each, revising and updating my book each year. During this period, classes of laboratory workers also asked for the course. Two physicians reviewed the book carefully and approved it.

It should be strongly emphasized that this book has been designed for the layman working in the field of medicine, including medical secretaries, physicians' assistants, medical claims adjustors, paramedical personnel, salesmen serving medical areas, and personnel associated with the health care industry. In other words, to aid those who work in all facets of the human health-care field to understand medical terms and how they apply to each of the body systems.

The book has been and can be used as a self-taught learning aid. The benefit any student receives will depend upon how much study is put into the subject. Body systems have been included to aid the student in relating the terms to parts of the body, but the emphasis should be on memorizing the terminology. The student should recognize that this book is in no way similar to a four-year premed course; what *can* be accomplished is an acquaintance with the language of medicine to the extent that the words have real meaning when encountered.

ACKNOWLEDGMENTS

Over the years this book was being written, revised, updated, and used, information was gathered from many sources — so many, in fact, I can't even remember them all. There are a few people, however, I'd like to mention and to whom I wish to express my gratitude.

Dr. Harvey S. Smith, an old-fashioned general practitioner, and his five sons, John, Robert, Richard, Harvey, and Carl, answered my questions and seeded my curiosity. My daughter, Barbara J. Rigsbee, CRNA, has been a constant source of information, advice, and encouragement; Dr. Maynard M. Conrad and Dr. Curtis M. Hanson helped me greatly to acquire knowledge of the musculoskeletal system; Dr. Fenimore T. Johnson reviewed the manuscript for correct usage and definitions of terms.

I extend my appreciation also to the authors of literally hundreds of texts I studied on anatomy, pathology, physiology, pharmacology, psychiatry, cardiology, and endocrinology, to name only a few fields.

Lastly, I would like to thank the more than one thousand students I have taught, who have kept me on my toes, pressured me for answers to their questions, and by their eagerness to acquire knowledge in the field of medical terminology, have helped to make this book what it is.

MEDICAL
TERMINOLOGY
AND THE
BODY
SYSTEMS

INTRODUCTION AND GUIDE TO STUDY

Medical terminology is the professional language of physicians and all others working in the field of medicine. It seems as complex as a foreign language at first, but as we discover *how* the terms are used and *why* they are used, learning becomes much easier.

Most medical terms are of Greek and Latin origin. Usually the name of an organ or part of the body is Latin, while the condition or disease affecting it is Greek. Some words come from French, such as *petit mal* and *malaise*. *Beriberi* comes from the Senegalese language. *Pellagra* is an Italian word. Other terms come from the German, Persian, Spanish, and Arabic languages. Medical terminology is thus a hybrid form of speech, a kind of jargon.

The pronunciation of terms follows no hard and fast rules. One might talk to three physicians in the same hospital and find that one will pronounce the word *gynecology* as "guy-nee-kology," another as "jinn-uh-kology," and a third as "jy-neh-kology."

Added to all this lexicographer's puzzle is the fact that in the study of medicine, the medical student must become familiar with the specialized language of several other branches of science: biology, chemistry, bacteriology, anatomy, endocrinology, pharmacology, and microbiology, to name only a few. The list of diseases, bacteria, drugs, and chemicals runs into the hundreds of thousands.

How are we to go about learning medical terminology? There is a relatively easy way. We will divide medical terms into their three components: prefixes (beginnings), roots (centers), and suffixes (endings).

Prefixes consist of one or more syllables carrying the clue to how many, or where, modifying the root: away from, toward, half, around, inside, both sides, above, below, etc.

Roots are the core of the term, describing the parts of the body affected: heart, liver, lungs, blood, bones, joints, etc.

Suffixes give the clue to the condition, disorder, or disease: inflammation, infection, rupture, stoppage, etc.

Let's see how this works by analyzing the term *endocarditis: endo* (prefix) = within; *card* (root) = heart; *itis* (suffix) = inflammation — in the layman's language, inflamation inside the heart.

Spelling is as important in medical terminology as knowledge of the meanings. For example, *adrenogenic* means originating in the adrenal glands; *androgenic* means originating from a male hormone. Obviously, the spelling vastly changes the meaning of the word.

STUDY TECHNIQUES

Within the past few years medical schools have discovered that by teaching medical terminology as it relates to the individual body systems, students learn more rapidly and retain more knowledge. This book has been designed along these lines, for that purpose.

There are specialties and specialists in every field of medicine. The guide which follows will show the reader where in this text to find the terms relating to each type of specialized medicine:

Allergists (specialists on allergies): **Integumentary** System and **Respiratory** System

Cardiologists (specialists on heart diseases): **Cardiovascular** and **Circulatory** Systems

Eye-Ear-Nose-Throat Specialists (self-explanatory): **Nervous** System

Gynecologists (specialists in women's diseases): **Reproductive** System

Internists (specialists in internal medicine): **Digestive, Excretory, Respiratory,** and **Endocrine** Systems

Neurologists (specialists in nervous diseases): **Nervous** System

Obstetricians (specialists for pregnancy): **Reproductive** System

Ophthalmologists (specialists in eye diseases): **Nervous** System

Orthopedists (bone and joint specialists): **Skeletal** and **Muscular** Systems

Pediatricians (baby specialists): All Systems

Psychiatrists (specialists in emotional disorders): All Systems

Urologists (specialists in urinary-tract disorders): **Urinary** System

Essentially this is a self-taught course. Learning terms is a vitally necessary process of drill and memorization, although much can be done to help the student relate to the terms.

Initially, read carefully through this Introduction and Guide to Study and look over the Glossaries. Do not attempt to learn all the terms in the Glossary when beginning the book. The Glossary is there to serve as a kind of minidictionary, to make it easy to look up a part of a term when the need arises. Note that a review test follows each of the first eight chapters.

Next, assign yourself one chapter at a time. Before studying each chapter, however, it is wise to become familiar with how the words studied in that chapter *sound*. Turn to the section of Pronunciations and Accents for Terms, and pronounce them *aloud* according to the phonetic spelling. (Then, when the chapter has been completed, go back and use that same section for further drill.) In this way, you will be able to understand the words and their meanings better. In addition, should you later be typing from a dictated tape, you will recognize the words.

Third, read the chapter. In memorizing terminology, one good way to learn the terms is to make a set of flash cards, writing the medical term on one side and the layman's term on the other. Then go through them looking at one side, calling out the term on the other. Routine drill will fix the prefixes, roots, suffixes and their various combinations in the mind. (The best approach to analysis of a term is to begin with the suffix and work backward to the root and prefix.)

Fourth, take the Review Test.

If you and a friend can study together, oral tests are excellent as an adjunct. Prepare a list of terms, a list of layman's descriptions of diseases or disorders which apply to the particular system, and questions pertaining to any extra reading material in the chapter; then quiz each other. Try to select terms *not* used in the written review test. For example, in the chapter on the Respiratory System, you might ask "What's ventilation? What's expiration? What's inspiration? What's diffusion? What's perfusion? How many lobes does the right lung have?" And so on.

Learn to look for any pertinent material in magazines, books, or other sources. Models of various parts of the body are also helpful, e.g., plastic models of the eye, the ear, or the brain.

Go to any source you can find — a doctor who is a personal friend, a friend who works in a hospital, and ask him to show you some medical instruments.

Another valuable aid is to obtain abstracts of medical papers on various diseases and their treatment. Pick out all the medical terms and define them. Medical Abstracts Services, a monthly publication by Physicians' Record Company, Berwyn, Illinois, is inexpensive, and one copy should provide several abstracts.

At the end of the first eight chapters there is a review test covering all the material studied up to that point. No review tests have been included for the chapters on Psychiatric Terminology and Pharmacology, since these two chapters are too broad for an ordinary test. The chapter on the Case History and Physical Examination Questionnaire is not meant to be memorized, but is included to show students who will be typing such forms for physicians what is usually included in this type of material. The 100-Question Prefinal Review should be taken just prior to the final examination. This comprehensive test will give the student a clear idea of where his weaknesses may lie so he can concentrate his study in that area.

If you are planning to work for a specialist, it is wise to learn all you can about the specialty — e.g., if you are planning to work for an orthopedic surgeon, go to the library and find whatever you can in books about the bones and joints, or ask the doctor himself to recommend a good book on the physiology of the musculoskeletal system. In the back of this book there is a list of recommended reading, with comments on the subject of each book, which may be helpful.

After you have completed this textbook, and are working in some field of medicine, you should search through a variety of medical journals, reading articles that apply to your particular field. Using this technique, you can continue to learn new terms related to your field of medicine.

ANATOMICAL SYSTEMS AND RELATED BODY PARTS

Respiratory

Nose, mouth, sinuses, larynx, pharynx, trachea, bronchi, lungs, pleura

Digestive and Excretory

Mouth, salivary glands, epiglottis, esophagus, cardia, stomach, liver, gallbladder, pylorus, duodenum, large and small intestines, ascending and descending colon, rectum, anus, spleen, pancreas

Skeletal and Muscular

Bones, joints, bursae, muscles, ligaments, tendons

Cardiovascular and Circulatory

Heart, arteries, veins, arterioles, venules, capillaries, blood

Nervous

Brain, spinal cord, nerves, peripheral and autonomous systems, sympathetic and parasympathetic systems, eyes and ears

Reproductive and Urinary (Genitourinary)

Female: uterus, ovaries, fallopian tubes, vagina, bladder, kidneys, urethra, ureter
Male: testes, penis, prostate, vas deferens, seminal vesicles, bladder, kidneys, urethra, ureter

Endocrine

Adrenals, pituitary, thyroids, parathyroids, pancreas, thymus, ovaries, testes, pineal gland

Integumentary

Dermis, epidermis, pores, sweat glands, sebaceous glands, hair, hair follicles, nails, epithelial tissue

PREFIXES, SUFFIXES, and ROOTS

From Medical to Laymen's Terms

a—, an—	without	cephalo—	head
ab—	away from	cera—	wax
ad—	toward	cerebro—	brain
aden—	gland	cervic—	neck
al—	like, similar	cheil—	lip
—algia	pain	cheir—,	
amyl—	starch	chiro—	hand
angio—	vessel (blood)	chole—	bile
ankyl—	crooked, looped	cholecyst	gallbladder
ante—	before	chondro—	cartilage
anti—	against	col—	colon
arterio—	artery	colp—	vagina
arthro—	joint	contra—	against
asthen—	weakness, lack	cort—	covering
aud—, aur—	ear, hearing	costo—	ribs
bar—	weight	cranio—	skull
bi—	both, two	—crine	secrete within
blepharo—	eyelid	cut—	skin
brachi—	arm	—cyesis	pregnancy
brady—	slow	cysto—	bladder, sac
bronchi—,		cyt—, cyte—	cell
broncho—	bronchial	dacry—	tear duct
bucca—	cheek	dactyl—	finger, toe
carcin—	cancer	—dema	swelling (fluid)
cardio—	heart	dent—	tooth
caud—	tail	derma—	skin
—cele	hernia	—desis	surgical fixation
—centesis	puncture	diplo—	double

dors—	back	*laryng—*	larynx
—duct	opening	*leuko—*	white
—dynia	pain	*lingua—*	tongue
dys—	painful, difficult	*lip—*	fat
—ectasis	enlargement	*lith—*	stone
ecto—	outside	*lymph—*	fluid
—ectomy	surgical removal	*—lysis*	separation
edem—	swelling (fluid)	*macro—*	large
—emia	blood	*—malacia*	softening
endo—	inside, within	*mamm—,*	
enter—	intestine	*mast—*	breast
epi—	upper, above	*—megaly*	enlarged
erythro—	red	*melan—*	black
faci—	facies, face	*mening—*	membrane
fascia	band (fibrous)	*meno—,*	
gastro—	stomach	*mens—*	menstruate
—genic	source, origin	*metro—*	uterus, womb
gingiva—	gums	*micro—*	small
gloss—	tongue	*mono—*	one, single
—gram,		*myelo—*	bone marrow
—graph	picture	*myo—*	muscle
gravid	pregnant	*myx—*	mucus
gyne—	woman	*nares—,*	
hemi—	half	*nas—*	nose, nostrils
hemo—	blood	*natus—*	birth
hepato—	liver	*nephro—*	kidney
hydro—	water	*neuro—*	nerve
hyper—	excessive	*ocul—*	eye
hypo—	deficient	*odont—*	tooth
hyster—	uterus, womb	*—oid*	like, similar
ile—	intestine (part)	*—ology*	study of
ili—	hip bone	*—olysis*	breakdown
inter—	between	*—oma*	tumor
intra—	inside	*onych—*	finger, toe nail
iri—	iris (eye)	*oophoro—*	ovary
—itis	inflammation	*ophthal—*	eye
kerat—	cornea; scaly	*orchis—*	testes
labia—	lip	*ortho—*	straight
lacto—	milk	*—osis*	disease, condition
lapar—	abdomen		(continued)

From Medical to Laymen's Terms (continued)

osteo—	bone	retro—	backward
—ostomy	surgical opening	rhin—	nose
oto—	ear, hearing	—rrhagia	hemorrhage
—otomy	incision	—rrhaphy	suture, stitch
ovario—	ovary	—rrhea	flowing
ovi—	egg	—rrhexis	rupture
pan—	all	salpingo—	tube
para—	beside	—sarcoma	tumor, cancer
part—	birth, labor	—sclerosis	hardening
—pathy	disease	—scope	picture, inspection
pĕd—, pōd—	foot	sebum	wax, suet
pēd—	child	semin—	seed
—penia	deficiency	sial—	saliva
peri—	around	soma—	body
—pexy	fixation (tissue)	—spasm	contraction
—phagia	swallow	splen—	spleen
pharyng—	pharynx	spondyl—	spine
—phasia	speak	squam—	scaly
phleb—	vein	—stasis	stoppage
—phobia	fear	stoma—	mouth
phren—	mind, diaphragm	stric—	narrowing
—physis	growth (physical)	sub—	below
—plasty	plastic surgery	super—	above
—plegia	paralysis	supra—	above
pleur—	pleura of lung	tachy—	rapid
pneumo—	lung	thel—	nipple
poly—	many	therm—	heat
post—	behind	thorac—	thorax
pre—	before	thrombo—	clot
pro—	forward	trache—	trachea
procto—	rectum	trachel—	neck
pseudo—	false	trans—	across
psycho—	mind, soul	—tripsy	crushing stone
—ptosis	dropping down	—uria	urine
pulm—	lung	vas—	vessel
pyelo—	bowl of kidney	vesic—	bladder, sac
pyo—	pus	viscera—	organ
ren—	kidney		

From Laymen's to Medical Terms

abdomen	*lapar—*	cornea	*kerat—*
above	*super—, supra—*	covering	*cort—*
across	*trans—*	crooked,	
against	*contra—*	looped	*ankyl—*
all	*pan—*	deficiency	*—penia*
arm	*brachi—*	deficient	*hypo—*
around	*peri—*	destruction	*—olysis*
away from	*ab—*	diaphragm,	
back	*post—*	mind	*phren—*
backward	*retro—*	difficult, painful	*dys—, dynia*
band	*fascia*	disease	*—osis, —pathy*
before	*ante—, pre—*	double	*diplo—*
behind	*post—*	dropping down	*—ptosis*
below	*sub—*	ear, hearing	*aud—, aur—, oto—*
beside	*para—*	enlargement	*—ectasis*
between	*inter—*	excessive,	
bile	*chole—*	extreme	*hyper—*
birth	*natus—, part—*	eye	*ophthalm—, ocul—*
black	*melan—*	eyelid	*blepharo—*
bladder	*cysto—*	face	*faci—*
blood	*hemo—, —emia*	false	*pseudo—*
body	*soma—*	fat	*lip—*
bone	*osteo—*	fear	*—phobia*
brain	*cerebro—*	finger	*—dactyl*
breakdown	*—olysis*	fixation	*—desis (bone only)*
breast	*mamm—, mast—*	fixation	*—pexy (tissue only)*
bronchial	*bronchi—, broncho—*	flow	*—rrhea*
cancer	*carcin—, sarcoma*	foot	*pĕd—, pōd—*
cartilage	*chondro—*	forward	*pro—*
cell	*cyt—, —cyte*	gallbladder	*cholecyst—*
cheek	*bucca—*	gland	*aden—*
chest	*thorac—*	growth	*—physis*
child	*ped—*	gums	*gingiva—*
closure	*stric—*	half	*hemi—*
clot	*thrombo—*	hand	*cheir—, chiro—*
colon	*col—*	hardening	*sclero—*
condition	*—osis*	head	*cephalo—*
contraction	*—spasm*		

(continued)

From Laymen's to Medical Terms (continued)

hearing	aud–, aur–	opening	
heart	cardio–	(permanent)	–ostomy
heat	therm–	opening	
hernia	–cele	(surgical)	–otomy
hip bone	ili–	opposite	contra–, anti–
horny, scaly	kerat–	organ	viscer–
incision	–otomy	origin, source	–genic
inflammation	–itis	outside	ecto–, exo–
inside	endo–, intra–	ovary	oophoro–
inspect	–scope	pain,	
intestine	enter–	painful	–algia, dys–
iris	iri–	paralysis	–plegia
joint	arthro–	pelvis (kidney)	–pyelo
kidney	nephro–	pharynx	pharyng–
labor	part–	picture	–gram, –graph
large	–megaly, –macro	plastic surgery	–plasty
larynx	laryng–	pleura	pleur–
like	–oid	pregnancy	–cyesis
lip	cheil–, labia	puncture,	
liver	hepato–	surgical	–centesis
lung	penumo–, pulm–	pus	pyo–
many	poly–	rapid	tachy–
marrow		rear, back	· post–
(bone)	myelo–	rectum	procto–
membrane	mening–	red	erythro–
menstruate	meno–, mens–	removal	
milk	lacto–	(surgical)	–ectomy
mind	psycho–	ribs	costo–
mouth	stoma–	rupture	–rrhexis
mucus	myx–	saliva	sial–
muscle	myo–	scaly	kerat–
nail	onych–	secrete	–crine
neck	trachel–, cervic–	seed	semin–
nerve	neuro–	similar, like	–oid
nipple	thel–	skin	derma–, cut–
nose	rhin–, nas–	skull	cranio–
one	mono–	slow	brady–
opening		small	micro–
(natural)	–duct		

softening	*—malacia*	tongue	*gloss—, lingua—*
source, origin	*—genic*	tooth	*odont—, dent—*
speak	*—phasia*	toward	*ad—*
spine	*spondyl—*	trachea	*trache—*
spleen	*splen—*	tube	*salpingo—*
starch	*amyl—*	tumor	*—oma*
stomach	*gastro—*	two, both	*bi—, duo—*
stone	*—lith*	upper	*epi—*
stone present	*lithiasis*	urine	*—uria*
stone crushing	*lithotripsy*	uterus	*hyster—, metro—*
stoppage	*—stasis*	vagina	*colp—*
straight	*ortho—*	vein	*phleb—*
study of	*—ology*	vertebra	*spondyl—*
suture	*—rrhaphy*	vessel	*angio—, vas—*
swallow	*—phagia*	water	*hydro—, lymph—*
swelling	*—dema*	wax	*cera—*
tail	*caud—*	weakness	*—asthenia*
tear duct	*dacry—*	weight	*bar—*
testicle	*orchis—*	white	*leuko—*
thorax	*thorac—*	without	*a—, an—*
toe, finger	*dactyl—*	woman	*gyne—*

COMMON ABBREVIATIONS

a.c.	before meals	**cath.**	catheterize
ACTH	adrenocortico-tropichormone	**cc**	cubic centimeter
ad lib	as desired	**CBC**	complete blood count
A—P	anterior—posterior (front & back)	**cm**	centimeter
A—P & lateral	anterior—posterior and side (as in x rays)	**CNS**	central nervous system
b.d., b.i.d.	twice a day	**CVA**	cerebrovascular accident (a "stroke")
b.m.	bowel movement	**D&C**	dilatation and currettage (of the uterus)
BMR	basal metabolism rate (a test)		
BUN	blood urea nitrogen (a test)	**DOA**	dead on arrival
		ECG, EKG	electrocardiogram (of the heart)
C	Centigrade temperature		

(continued)

COMMON ABBREVIATIONS (continued)

EEG	electroencephalo-gram (of the brain)	**IPPB**	intermittent positive-pressure breathing
EENT	eye—ear—nose and throat	**I.V.**	intravenously (liquid fed into a vein)
E.R.	emergency room		
ESR	erythrocyte sedi-mentation rate		
EST	electroshock therapy (for mental patients)	**LD$_{50}$**	lethal dose for 50% of test animals
		mg	milligram
F	Fahrenheit temperature	ml	milliliter
		mm	millimeter
F.B.S.	fasting blood sugar (a test)	**n—p**	neuropsychiatric
		N.P.O.	nothing by mouth
G-I	gastrointestinal	**OB**	obstetrics
gm	gram		
gr	grain	**O.R.**	operating room
G-U	genitourinary	**OTC**	over the counter (as refers to drugs)
Hct	hematocrit (usually as refers to a blood test)	**P.A.R.**	postanesthesia recovery ("the recovery room")
h.d., h.s.	taken at bedtime		
Hgb	hemoglobin (usually as refers to a blood test)	**p.c.**	after meals
		P.E.	physical examination
I.C.U.	intensive care unit		
I.M.	intramuscularly (injection)	**pH**	symbol for measuring degree of acidity
I&O	intake and output (liquid drunk and urine output)	**P.H.**	past history (case history)

p.r.n.	whenever necessary	**T&A**	tonsillectomy and adenoidectomy
pt.	patient	**t.d.s., t.i.d.**	three times a day
q.d.	every day	**T.L.C.**	tender loving care
q.i.d.	four times a day	**TPR**	temperature, pulse, and respiration
q.q.h., q.4 h.	every four hours		
q.s.	in sufficient quantity	**U.R.I.**	upper respiratory infection
RBC	red blood cell count	**U.S.P.**	United States Pharmacopeia
STAT	anything which must be done *immediately*	**U.T.I.**	urinary tract infection
		V.C.	vital capacity
T.A.	tetanus antitoxin	**v.d.**	venereal disease
T.A.T.	thematic apperception test	**WBC**	white blood cell count

THE RESPIRATORY SYSTEM

As we trace the route of the respiratory system, please compare the numbers on this page with those in the line drawing in Fig. 1.

1. The *respiratory center,* which sends messages to the lungs to inhale, is located in the brain.
2. The *frontal sinuses* are located above the eyes on each side of the forehead. All eight sinuses help keep air pressure in the nasal cavity fairly equal, and control to some extent the tone of the voice, giving it more or less depth of tonal quality.
3. The *sphenoid sinuses* are located back of the nose.
4. The *ethmoid sinuses* lie slightly below each eye.
5. The *nasal cavity* allows the air we breathe to be filtered and warmed.
6. The *mouth* gives us another airway, and also moistens and warms the air we breathe.
7. The *maxillary sinuses* lie within each cheek bone.
8. The *tonsils* are located on each side of the back of the throat.
9. The *pharynx* is the tissue that lines the back of the nose, mouth, and throat.
10. The *larynx* is the "voice box," helping, along with the vocal cords, to produce speech. The vocal cords vibrate with the outward flow of air; their tension determines to some extent the pitch and tone of voice, which is also influenced by the muscles of the larynx. The "Adam's Apple" is the cartilage covering of the larynx.

11. The *trachea,* or windpipe, is lined with mucous membrane covered with *cilia* (tiny fine hairs) which continuously sweep foreign particles out of the breathing passages up to the mouth.
12. The trachea branches at its end and leads into the *bronchi,* or bronchial tubes.
13. The *pleura* are double-walled membranes enclosing each lung.
14. The *lungs* do the real work of the respiratory system by giving the oxygen we breathe in to the red blood cells. Lung tissue can be stretched or expanded. The lung can also be collapsed for some types of surgery. The left lung is smaller than the right, to accommodate the heart.
15. The *bronchioles* are finer "branches" of the "bronchial tree."
16. The *alveoli* are microscopic, balloon-shaped clusters throughout the lungs. When filled with air, the lungs look like sponges do when they are filled with water.

The respiratory center in the brain responds to any increase of carbon dioxide in the body. When the level of carbon dioxide reaches a certain point, this center sends a message to the lungs to inhale. If the brain has been damaged, the lungs will, in some circumstances, take over on their own and cause the respiratory cycle to continue.

With *inspiration* (inhalation), the diaphragm (the membrane separating the stomach and chest) flattens downward and the muscles between the ribs (*intercostal* muscles) cause the rib cage to flare out at the bottom, creating an increase in the capacity of the *thorax* (the chest). Air is pulled in, and the alveoli fill with air. When they are full, a reflex stops inhalation and starts *expiration* (exhalation). Air is forced out of the lungs, carrying the carbon dioxide residue. We take in much more oxygen than we use, to aid in removing carbon dioxide. The air we normally breathe is about 20% oxygen.

The four phases of respiration are: *ventilation,* passage of air into the bronchi; *distribution* of air to all parts of the lungs; *diffusion,* the spreading of air into the alveoli; and *perfusion,* as oxygen is absorbed by the blood and carbon dioxide is given off.

Each lung is enclosed in a double-walled membrane called the *pleura.* These walls may become inflamed during a cold or pneumonia; the serum, or fluid, between the two membranes is then exuded, causing discomfort or pain.

Lung tissue expands and contracts much like a bellows during the respiratory cycle. The right lung has three lobes: the superior (top),

THE RESPIRATORY SYSTEM

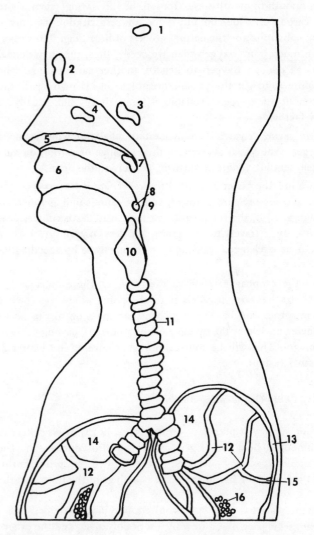

Figure 1

middle, and inferior (bottom), while the left lung has only two lobes, superior and inferior. Each lobe is subdivided into six segments separated by connective tissue. The right lung has three branches of the bronchial tree, while the left lung has only two branches.

Four questions are frequently asked regarding the respiratory system:

1. How can mouth-to-mouth resuscitation be life-saving when we're exhaling carbon dioxide? Mouth-to-mouth resuscitation is only a temporary substitute for the natural process of breathing. Remember, we take in much more oxygen than we need; thus, the air we exhale still contains enough oxygen to benefit another pair of lungs. The main purpose is to get the patient breathing on his own again; the actual amount of oxygen available is, not always but usually, a secondary factor.

2. Why do we yawn? A yawn is an involuntary inhalation when we need more oxygen. The yawn accelerates the exchange of carbon dioxide and oxygen, sending a more stimulating mixture to the brain.

3. Why do we breathe faster at high altitudes? There is less oxygen the higher we get, air pressure is lower, and we cannot pull as much air into the lungs. Also, the temperature at high altitudes is colder; air is warmed less as it travels to the lungs; and less oxygen and carbon dioxide can be exchanged, causing us to compensate by speeding up inhalation.

4. How does the esophagus relate to the trachea? The esophagus lies behind the trachea and parallels it to the point where the trachea branches into the bronchi. The esophagus continues on to the *cardia* (the sphincter muscle at the opening of the stomach), passing through the diaphragm. This will be more thoroughly covered in Chapter 2, The Digestive System.

The Heart-Lung Pump-Oxygenating Machine

When major surgery is necessary on the lungs, heart, or elsewhere in the chest, a bloodless field for surgery makes the procedure easier. The heart-lung pump-oxygenating machine was designed to provide this bloodless field by diverting blood from the chambers of the heart and the lungs.

The human heart has two synchronized pumping systems: one a valvular system, regulating blood flow by a series of valves, and the other a propulsion system, operated by the heart muscles. The lungs are a pair of bellows which fill and empty 15 to 25 times a minute. Their primary function is to remove carbon dioxide from venous blood and put oxygen into arterial blood. When they fail to function, the result is cardiorespiratory failure. The heart-lung pump-oxygenator makes it possible to bypass the heart and lungs, while still maintaining respiration and circulation. Respiration is continued by "bag-breathing," which the anesthetist does by manually operating a plastic bag, forcing air into and out of the lungs. The machine removes blood from the superior and inferior vena cava (see drawing of the heart in Fig. 4.), feeds oxygen into the blood, and pumps it back into the arteries at exactly the same rate as the patient's normal circulation. This is necessary because blood pressure must be maintained at a normal level during surgery.

Body temperature can be reduced by means of a temperature control mechanism in the machine. Hypothermia, lowering body temperature by use of ice packs or refrigerating blankets, may also be used. Lowered body temperature creates a slower rate of blood circulation – an advantage in this type of surgery.

The machine must be placed 18 to 24 inches below the level of the patient's heart. Monitoring instruments measure oxygen content of the blood, its temperature, carbon dioxide content, blood pressure, and blood volume. The machine must be free of any material which would have a chemical or toxic effect on the circulating blood. Newer plastics such as polyethylene are best for this purpose and seem to inhibit clotting while the blood is outside the patient's body. The oxygenator "bubbles" oxygen into the blood by forcing the oxygen through two extremely thin membranes of teflon, while thin sheets of blood are pumped between them. The blood absorbs the oxygen as it passes through.

Most large hospitals now have these machines, which are about the size of large refrigerators and can be moved about on wheels.

DISEASES AND DISORDERS

Adenoiditis. *Aden–* means gland; *–oid* means like. Adenoids are glandlike tissue, located at the back of the nasopharyngeal area. Adenoiditis is inflammation of this adenoidal tissue, and is most common in young children. When tonsils are removed, adenoids are usually removed also.

Allergies. While allergic reactions affect other parts of the body, they attack the respiratory system severely at times. Allergies can be caused by foods, pollens, dust, molds, animal hair, grasses, and emotional problems, among other things. The mucous membranes of the nose, mouth, and throat are irritated, causing inflammation, edema, and swelling. Excessive amounts of *histamine* are released, dilating the capillaries and stimulating production of fluid and mucus. Allergies also attack the skin, eyes, heart, and nervous system. Antihistamine medications are given to relieve the symptoms, and sometimes, if the allergic reaction is severe, steroids may be given.

Asthma. This can be a rather serious disorder, resulting in inflammation and constriction of the bronchial mucosa (mucous lining of the bronchial tubes). In the asthmatic patient, normal tissue of the bronchi has been damaged due to repeated attacks. When an asthmatic gasps, wheezes, chokes, and coughs, further damage occurs. Chronic asthma leads to infection, and infection brings more prolonged serious attacks. The violence of the coughing breaks down delicate tissue of the alveoli, and the patient's life span is shortened. Rehabilitation requires rest, proper diet, no smoking, and the use of bronchodilators.

Bronchitis. Inflammation of the bronchial tubes, frequently accompanied by a "dry" unproductive cough. If there is infection present also, the cough is "bubbly" and productive of mucus. Antibiotics may be given if there is bacterial infection.

Common colds. Disorders of the upper respiratory tract with a runny nose, watery eyes, coughing, sneezing, and sometimes with chills and fever. It is believed that colds are caused by a virus. The best treatment is bed rest, aspirin, and plenty of fluids.

Emphysema. This disease created by some irritant to the bronchi and lungs, causes the lungs to become permanently distended and often covered with scar tissue. The lungs lose their ability to contract, so the patient is continually trying to expand his lungs even more. The alveoli eventually fill with fibrous tissue. Emphysema is characterized by shortness of breath and a chronic cough.

Empyema. Accumulation of pus in a body cavity, in this case the chest, in either the lungs or the pleura or both. The disease may start after an attack of pneumonia or pleurisy. There is likely to be fever, loss of strength, loss of weight, and painful or difficult breathing.

Influenza. An acute, infectious, epidemic disease marked by fever, chills, acute inflammation of the nose, throat, and bronchi, with muscular pain and often gastrointestinal disorders. There are many types, and the virus seems to be able to change from year to year; thus we have "Asian Flu," "Hong Kong," and many other varieties. Complications involving the respiratory system are frequent.

Laryngitis. Inflammation of the larynx, with difficulty in both speaking and swallowing; sometimes accompanied by a cold or cough.

Mastoiditis. Inflammation and usually infection of the mastoid area in the temporal bone of the skull, most often in the area behind the ear.

Otitis media. Inflammation, and often infection, of the middle ear.

Pharyngitis. Inflammation of the pharynx, involving the walls of the nose, mouth, and throat. As in laryngitis, there usually is difficulty in speaking and swallowing.

Pleurisy. The membranous coverings of the lungs become inflamed and painful when a breath is taken. "Dry" pleurisy is accompanied by a frictional rubbing of the inner and outer pleural membranes, causing shallow breathing. "Serofibrinous" pleurisy is accompanied by exudate from the pleura. Sometimes this fluid must be aspirated (drawn off or suctioned out) for relief of the condition.

Pneumonia, bronchial. An inflammation and infection of the lungs which usually begins in the bronchioles — often follows infections of the upper respiratory tract.

Pneumonia, lobar. An acute lung disease marked by inflammation and infection of one or more lobes of the lungs, attended by chills, fever, rapid breathing, cough, and pain in the chest.

Pneumonitis. A localized inflammation of the lung — usually a "benign" type of pneumonia.

Pulmonary tuberculosis. Caused by inhalation of tubercle bacilli which results in involvement of the lungs, bronchi, pleura, and the pulmonary lymph nodes. Lesions appear in the lungs, but may become arrested and heal, leaving scar tissue. Once a widespread disease, tuberculosis is now treated successfully with antibiotics.

Sinusitis. Inflammation of any or all of the sinus cavities in the head, frequently resulting in sinus infections and drainage of purulent material (pus).

Tonsillitis. Inflamed tonsils, usually with accompanying infection.

Tracheitis. Inflammation of the trachea, accompanied by cough and hoarseness.

Combined forms. Tonsillopharyngitis, tracheobronchitis, otolaryngitis, tracheopharyngitis.

TERMINOLOGY

The combining of roots and suffixes, or of prefixes and roots, or of all three — prefixes, roots, and suffixes — will be puzzling to the new student of terminology because of the change in vowels when the three are put together. For example, when *bronchi−* is combined with *−itis*, the "i" at the end of *bronchi* is dropped, so that the word is not *bronchiitis* but *bronchitis.* However, this is not a rule without exceptions. Note that the word *bronchiectasis* leaves the "i" in *bronchi−* to go along with the "e" in *−ectasis.*

While the root for lips is *labia−*, almost always the last "a" in the root changes to an "o," as in *labioplasty.* This change really denotes that the term is a *combined* form. The only true method for correctly spelling the terms is to memorize them. If the student, in his work, encounters a new term he has not yet learned, it is wise to look it up in a medical dictionary to be sure of the correct spelling. Generally, when terms are combined and two vowels come together, one of the vowels is dropped. But remember that this is not always true. In some cases, when two vowels fall together in combining the terms, a letter is *added;* for example, the term for mouth is *stoma,* but a "t" is added for *stomatitis* and *stomatoma.*

Roots	Terms	Descriptions
aud−, aur−	auditory nerve	nerve controlling hearing
oto−	ot/itis media	infection, inflammation of the middle ear
ear, hearing	oto/laryng/itis	inflammation of ear & larynx
bronchi−	bronch/itis	inflammation of the bronchial tubes
broncho−	bronchi/ectasis	enlargement, dilation of the bronchi
bronchus	broncho/genic	originating within the bronchial tubes

Roots	Terms	Descriptions
cheil—	cheilo/sarcoma	tumor or cancer of the lip
labia—	labio/plasty	plastic surgery on the lips
lips	labio/rrhaphy	suturing the lip
costo—	costo/chondral	pertaining to ribs and cartilage
ribs	inter/costal	between the ribs
gloss—	gloss/itis	inflammation of the tongue
lingua—	lingua/lithiasis	stone in or under tongue
tongue	sub/lingual	beneath or below the tongue
laryng—	laryng/ectomy	surgical removal of larynx
larynx	laryngo/scope	inspection of the larynx
pharyng—	pharyngo/spasm	spasmodic contraction of the pharynx
pharynx	pharyng/itis	inflammation of the pharynx
pleur—	pleura/centesis	surgical puncture of the pleura
pleura	pleuro/dynia	pain in the pleura
pneumo—	pneumon/ectomy	surgical removal of a lung
	pneumon/olysis	breakdown of lung tissue
pulm—	pulmonary edema	fluid, swelling of lungs
lung		
naris—	nares	the nostrils
nas—	naso/plasty	plastic surgery on the nose
rhin—	rhino/rrhea	running nose
nose	naso/pharyngeal	nasal area of the pharynx
stoma	stomat/itis	inflammation in the mouth
mouth	stomat/oma	tumor of the mouth
thorac—	thorac/otomy	incision into the chest
chest	pneumo/thoracic	lung area of the chest
trache—	tracheo/rrhexis	rupture of the trachea
trachea	trache/otomy	incision into the trachea
cervic —	cervical spine	portion of spine at the neck
trachel—	trachel/osis	disease of the neck
neck	trachel/oma	tumor of the neck

You have also learned a number of suffixes combined with the above roots:

—*centesis*	surgical puncture
—*dynia*	pain
—*ectasis*	enlargement, dilation
—*ectomy*	surgical removal
—*genic*	source or origin
—*itis*	inflammation
—*lithiasis*	presence of stones
—*olysis*	breakdown (of tissue or cells)
—*oma*	tumor
—*osis*	disease or condition
—*otomy*	surgical incision
—*plasty*	plastic surgery
—*rrhaphy*	suturing or stitching
—*rrhea*	running, flowing
—*rrhexis*	rupture
—*sarcoma*	malignant tumor or cancer
—*scope*	picture or inspection

Additional Vocabulary

acute: severe right now; critical (compare with chronic)

anoxia: lack of oxygen in body tissues (compare with hypoxia)

apnea: no visible breathing (compare with dyspnea, tachypnea)

aspirate: to draw out, as aspirating fluid from the pleura

auscultation: listening to sounds in the body (see palpation)

bronchoconstrictor: medication causing constriction of bronchi

bronchodilator: medication to dilate lung's air passages

chronic: long-lasting, recurrent, as in chronic bronchitis

cilia: tiny hairs attached to free surface of cells

(continued)

Additional Vocabulary (continued)

diaphragm: a membranous wall between the chest and stomach

dysphagia:* painful or difficult swallowing

dysphasia:* painful or difficult speaking, as in stuttering

dyspnea: painful or difficult breathing

E.E.N.T.: eye-ear-nose-throat (or E.N.T.: ear-nose-throat)

epistaxis: nosebleed

extrinsic: originating outside the body, as in extrinsic allergy

hypoxia: lack of oxygen in the air being breathed

intrinsic: originating within the body, as in intrinsic asthma

mucous: adjective describing secretion from moist membranes

mucus: fluid secretion from moist membranes of the body

oral: pertaining to the mouth, as in oral medication

parenteral: injected medication, intramuscular or intravenous

palpation: pressing the body to feel the shape of an organ

percussion: striking with short blows, as percussing the chest

rales: musical rattling or bubbling sounds in the chest, bronchi

resonant: vibrant, echoing sounds in the chest

sibilant: whispering, murmuring sounds in the chest

sonorous: deep booming sounds in the chest

tachypnea: excessively rapid breathing

U.R.I.: upper respiratory infection

* To help the student in remembering the difference between *dysphasia* and *dysphagia*, fix in your mind that *dysphasia* has an "s" and relate it to *speaking*, while *dysphagia* has a "g" and relate it to *gulp* — which is a kind of swallowing. Any such tricks the student can think of to relate to terms will be helpful in memorization.

*Pronunciations and Accents
for Terms**

alveoli	al-vee'-oh-lee
anoxia	an-knock'-see-uh
antigen	ant'-eh-jen
auscultation	aws-cul-tay'-shun
bronchi	bron'-kee
bronchial	bron'-kee-al
bronchiectasis	bron-kee-ek'-tasis
bronchiole	bron'-kee-ole
bronchogenic	bron-ko-jen'-ik
cervical	ser'-vik-al
cheilosarcoma	kyle-oh-sar-ko'ma
cilia	sil'-ee-ah
costochondral	cost-oh-kon'-dral
diaphragm	dye'-uh-fram
dysphagia	dis-fay'-jee-ah
dysphasia	dis-fay'-see-ah
dyspnea	dis'-pnee-ah
edema	eh-dee'-mah
emphysema	em-fa-see'-mah
empyema	em-pie-ee'-mah
epistaxis	ep-eh-stack'-sis
esophagus	ee-sof'-uh-gus
ethmoid	eth'-moyd
glossitis*	gloss-eye'-tis
histamine	his'-tuh-meen
hypothermia	high-po-ther'-mee-ah
hypoxia	high-pock'-see-ah
labioplasty	lay'-bee-oh-plasty
labiorrhaphy	lay-bee-oh'-raf-ee
laryngectomy	lair-in-jek'-toe-mee
laryngoscope	lair-in'-joe-skope
larynx	lair'inks (*not* lair-nix)
lingualithiasis	ling-wah-lith-eye'-uh-sis
mastoiditis*	mass-toy-die'-tis
nares	nair'-eez

nasopharynx	nay-zo-fair´-inks
otitis media	oh-tie´-tis mee´-dee-ah
otolaryngitis *	oh-toe-lair-in-jy´-tis
parenteral	pair-en´-ter-al
pharynx	fair´-inks (*not* fair-nix)
pharyngospasm	fair-in´-joe-spasm
pineal	pin´-ee-all
pleura	ploo´-rah
pleurisy	ploo´-reh-see
pleurodynia	ploo-row-din´-ee-ah
pneumocentesis	new-moe-sen-tee´-sis
pneumonectomy	new-moe-neck´-toe-me
pneumonitis *	new-moe-nigh´-tis
pneumonolysis	neo-moe-noll´-eh-sis
pneumosarcoma	new-moe-sar-ko´-mah
pneumothoracic	new-moe-tho-rass´-ik
rales	ralls
rhinoplasty	rine´-oh-plas-tee
rhinorrhea	rine-oh-ree´-ah
serofibrinous	seer-oh-fy´-brin-us
sibilant	sib´-eh-lant
sphenoid	sfee´-noyd
sphincter	sfink´-ter
thoracic	tho-rass´-ik
thoracotomy	tho-rah-kot´-oh-mee
trachea	tray´-kee-ah
tracheitis *	tray-kee-eye´-tis
tracheloma	tray-kel-oh´-mah
trachelosis	tray-kel-oh´-sis
tracheorrhexis	tray-kee-oh-rex´-us
tracheospasm	tray-´ kee-oh-spasm
tracheotomy	tray-kee-ott´-oh-me
vena cava	vee´-na kay´-vah
venous	vee´-nuss

* While the American way of pronouncing *—itis* is "eye-tiss," British doctors and many foreign doctors practicing in the United States pronounce the suffix as "eee-tis." The meaning and correct spelling remain the same.

REVIEW TEST: THE RESPIRATORY SYSTEM

1. Where is the respiratory center located?

2. Which lung is the larger?   Why?

3. Name five disorders or diseases of the respiratory system.

4. Define alveoli.

5. Define tracheotomy.

6. Define stomatitis.

7. Define tracheorrhexis.

8. Define tracheloma.

9. Give term for puncture of lung.

10. Give term for stone under tongue.

11. Give term for pain in pleura.

12. Give term for removal of a lung.

13. Give term for incision in chest.

14. Give term for cancer of the lip.

15. Differentiate between dysphasia and dysphagia.

16. Differentiate between emphysema and empyema.

17. Differentiate between laryngotomy and laryngectomy.

18. Differentiate between laryngitis and pharyngitis.

19. Differentiate between bronchitis and bronchiectasis.

20. Define rhinorrhea.

THE DIGESTIVE AND EXCRETORY SYSTEM

Trace the route of the digestive and excretory systems by comparing the following descriptions with Figure 2.

1. The *mouth* is the beginning of the digestive system, where food mixes with saliva and some digestive juices while it is being chewed.

2. The *salivary glands* lubricate the mouth and make food easier to chew and swallow. There are six, three on each side of the mouth. These are controlled by the nervous system.

3. The *epiglottis*, which opens when we swallow, is a lidlike covering made of cartilage.

4. The *esophagus* (gullet) extends from the pharynx to the stomach.

5. The *cardia* is a sphincter muscle at the upper opening of the stomach. The cardia is open when the stomach is empty, and closed while food is being digested.

6. The *stomach* is where food is mixed with bile, acids, and enzymes to aid in digestion.

7. The *pylorus* is a sphincter muscle at the bottom opening of the stomach, which opens to allow food to enter the intestines.

8. The *duodenum* is the first part of the small intestine.

9. The *small intestine* is a mass of coiled tubing where the digestive process is almost completed in the *jejunum* and *ileum*.

10. The *ascending colon* carries the molecules of nutritional material upward, and these molecules begin to be absorbed by the body.

11. The *transverse colon* travels across the body, continuing the absorptive process and carrying waste material along.

12. The *descending colon* is the area where waste matter resulting from digestion enters the excretory system.

13. The *appendix* is an appendage or pouch off the ascending colon.

14. The *rectum* is where waste material lies until contractions create a desire to move the bowels.

15. The *anus* is the terminal opening of the alimentary canal.

Thus, the digestive and excretory systems can be pictured as one long tube extending from the mouth to the anus. It is characterized by its moist inner surface containing millions of tiny glands producing mucus and enzymes to break down foods. This tube has a relatively thick muscular wall which is involved in mixing, churning, and moving.

The digestive system is a chemical plant, working on food the moment you put it in your mouth. Food begins to break down as it is chewed, mixing with *ptyalin,* an enzyme secreted by the salivary glands, which begins at once the conversion of carbohydrates or starches into sugar.

Muscular action of the tract, or peristalsis, keeps the mixture moving. Upon swallowing — a muscular action in itself — food is moved down the esophagus. At each swallow the epiglottis, a lidlike covering of cartilage, opens and the food enters the esophagus. Three to five seconds later, another muscular contraction sends food through the cardia to the stomach, a receiving station that pours into the mixture such chemicals as hydrochloric acid, pepsin, rennin, lipase, acids, enzymes, and other secretions. There are over 35 million glands in the stomach alone.

The cardia, a sphincter muscle at the upper opening of the stomach, closes when food is being digested but opens with each peristaltic wave. When the stomach has finished its part of the digestive process, another sphincter muscle at the lower end of the stomach, the pylorus, opens and contractions become stronger as the food enters the duodenum, so called because it is usually 12 fingers long: *duo* = 2, plus *denum* = 10.

Liquids pass rapidly through the digestive tract, but solid foods lie in the stomach several hours before liquefying enough to pass on. The semiliquid state of food after mixing with gastric juices is called *chyme*.

The small intestine is lined with tiny budlike projections called *villi* (fine hairs), and through these the food substances are absorbed into the blood stream, molecule by molecule, as they are separated from the waste

THE DIGESTIVE AND EXCRETORY SYSTEMS

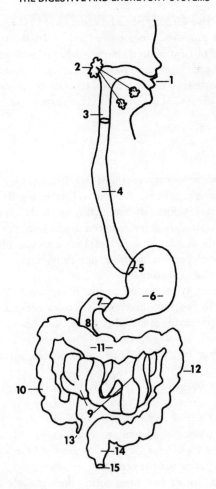

Figure 2

material. There are about 5 million villi; if the small intestine could be spread out in one continuous flat surface, there would be an absorptive area of 100 square feet — almost as large as a 9-by-12 rug.

Proteins and carbohydrates are partially digested in the duodenum, but fats show little change. Progress through the 20 feet of small intestine is slow, taking 3 to 5 hours. Intestinal muscles move, mix, and churn food much as a screw-type food grinder performs. The mixture passes from the small intestine to the ascending colon, through the transverse colon to the descending colon.

The colon is inactive for long periods. When food has been thoroughly processed, a reflex is produced when more food enters the stomach. This reflex causes a wave of contractions, moving what is now waste material into the colon and upper rectum. Rectal pressure rises, and powerful contractions of these muscles create a desire to move the bowels. The anus sphincter muscle is controlled by the will. The waste products are called *feces*, or fecal matter.

The Liver

Since the liver is one organ we cannot live without, we need to know something about how it functions. The liver is located on the right side of the upper abdomen and is dome-shaped, fitting under the rib cage. Its size is constant in good health, weighing between 2 and 3 pounds in the male, and slightly less in the female. It is reddish-brown to chocolate in color, with an undersurface of deep indigo blue, due to liberation of iron in the pigment. It is a soft solid in texture.

The liver is a strangely misleading organ: In structure, it seems to be one of the simplest. In function, however, it is most complex. Liver cells all look alike, and apparently each cell is a jack-of-all-trades — for it can take in, build up, break down, and cast off. The liver has a unique power of repair, so that if part of the liver is damaged or removed it can rebuild itself to a degree.

The liver is also unique in that 80% of the blood it receives comes from the *portal veins*. As a result, liver cells are peculiarly liable to *necrosis* (death) from *anoxia* (lack of oxygen), but the *hepatic artery* maintains an oxygen tension that usually overcomes this danger. There are great variations in the volume of blood flowing through the lobes of the liver; it never works at full capacity but has great reserve power.

The liver is made up of two main lobes, the right lobe being about twice the size of the left. The gallbladder lies just below and behind the center of the right lobe. Blood from the stomach and the spleen enter the left lobe, while the right lobe obtains blood from the duodenum and pancreas. Mysteriously, there is little intermingling of these two blood streams.

The liver plays a vital role in nutrition and maintenance of the body, for it dominates metabolism of food. Extracts from food are conveyed from the intestines to the liver, which then functions as a master cook in making the food usable. It has been called a chemical factory, a receiving depot, and a storehouse.

Bile is manufactured in the liver, passes through the gallbladder to the bile duct, and thence into the digestive system. The liver turns *glycogen* (animal starch) into *glucose* (sugar), which is as necessary to life as oxygen, for it is consumed constantly by the body cells. The liver regulates protein metabolism, turning proteins into amino acids; it regulates fat metabolism, manufactures ketones, and forms plasma proteins. The synthesis of serum albumin, prothrombin, and fibrinogen is accomplished in the liver. Without fibrinogen there would be faulty blood coagulation. Male and female sex hormones are shunted to the liver, processed, excreted in the bile, and reabsorbed by the body. The body's absorption of vitamin K depends largely upon the liver.

The Spleen

For nearly 2000 years the spleen was considered an organ of mystery, and still is to some extent. Until about 20 years ago it was believed that life could not be maintained without the spleen, but with the great increase in automobile accidents, many spleens have been ruptured or damaged beyond repair and have had to be removed. Yet the patients have lived. The mystery is how one of the most vital body organs can be removed without any drastic change in vitality.

The spleen is located at the back of the abdomen, opposite the liver and adjacent to the pancreas. Its average weight is a little less than half a pound, its color is reddish-purple, similar to the liver, and it is a rather soft mass which pulsates and contains some muscular tissue. Unlike the liver, pancreas, and kidneys, the spleen is an abdominal organ without a duct. However, it is not a ductless gland; it's like a sponge, designed to retain and alter the blood which filters through it. Its functions apparently are to *produce* blood, to *purify* blood, to act as a *reservoir* for blood, and to *destroy* useless parts of the blood. Its complete function is still not known; nor have scientists yet learned whether the circulation of blood through the spleen is an "open" or "closed" type circulation process.

Blood production. Before birth, blood elements are produced in the spleen. After birth, the bone marrow takes over this job, but if bone marrow function is affected by some disease, the spleen will again begin production. It is believed the spleen controls bone marrow blood production, but the relationship is not yet known.

Blood purification. Blood enters the spleen on the venous side through a sphincter muscle and seems to be filtered through the tissues. When the spleen is filled, the sphincters on both the venous and arterial sides close and the blood remains inside the spleen for varying periods of time, sometimes as long as 10 hours. During this period, erythrocytes and plasma are changed so they are more readily absorbable and usable. Then the sphincter muscle on the arterial side opens, and the blood passes back into general circulation.

Blood reservoir. The spleen is sometimes called a "blood bank," because it can store a large supply of blood or empty itself instantly when there is a sudden demand from the body, such as a hemorrhage.

Blood destruction. The spleen removes from the blood those parts which are old, useless, damaged, or deteriorated. This is particularly true of red blood cells. The spleen is called the graveyard of erythrocytes. Abnormal cells such as those which cause leukemia, sickle cell anemia, and hemolytic anemia are usually trapped and destroyed in the spleen.

Although people can live without a spleen, we know they are much more susceptible to various blood diseases when the organ has been removed. Typhoid fever, malaria, tuberculosis, and syphilis enlarge the spleen. Tumors and cancers of the spleen are relatively rare, perhaps because of the purifying process that takes place within it.

The Pancreas

The pancreas is a gland secreting powerful digestive juices, and is also an endocrine gland, one of the chief regulators of carbohydrate metabolism. This organ arises as a "bud" from the intestinal canal, its opening entering the duodenum at about the same point as the common bile duct. Scattered throughout the pancreas are the tiny islets discovered by Dr. Langerhans in 1869 and bearing his name — the islets of

Langerhans. These represent the endocrine element, which manufactures alpha and beta cells. The beta cells produce insulin, while the alpha cells manufacture glycogen.

The pancreas secretes from about 1 cup to 1 pint of fluid every 24 hours. This fluid contains insulin, glucagon, and three powerful digestive enzymes — trypsin, amylase, and lipase. Trypsin breaks down proteins, amylase converts starches to a malt, and lipase splits fats into glycerol and free fatty acids. Insulin is vital to body health. It is secreted into the blood where it regulates carbohydrate (sugar) metabolism. Without insulin the amount of sugar in the blood increases, and this in turn causes something to go wrong with our utilization of fats. Sugar cannot be stored, so it passes off in the urine.

DISEASES AND DISORDERS

Appendicitis. An inflamed appendix. If infection is present, this usually requires surgical removal of the appendix.

Cardiaspasm. A spasm of the cardia, the sphincter muscle at the upper opening to the stomach, and not connected with the heart at all, although the symptoms are intense pain in the region of the heart, causing the patient anxiety that he is having a heart attack. Cause is unknown. Antispasmodics are helpful.

Cholecystitis. Inflammation of the gallbladder, usually caused by one or more gallstones. The stones may be removed, leaving the gallbladder, but more often the entire gallbladder is removed.

Colitis, mucous or spastic. Inflammation of the colon with spasmodic contractions and the passage of mucus when the bowels move. Cure demands a mild diet, no alcohol, plenty of rest, and often tranquilizers. Tension, rebellion, and emotional repression are causes.

Colitis, ulcerative. A grave disorder involving chronic ulcers in the colon. This type is very difficult to cure.

Constipation. May be caused by an organic disorder such as an intestinal obstruction, or may be functional, caused by lack of enough roughage and liquids in the diet.

Diarrhea. An abnormal liquid consistency of the bowels, accompanied by an abnormal frequency of bowel movements. This may be a symptom of an organic digestive tract disorder, or may be caused by food poisoning.

Diverticulitis. Inflammation of the diverticula of the intestine, with herniated pouches or defective sites in the muscular wall of the intestine. Fecal matter collects in these pouches, causing severe pain and infection. Surgery to remove parts of the intestine may be necessary.

Dysentery. There are two forms: amebic, caused by eating or drinking a substance containing amebae, and bacillary, caused by bacteria of the Shigella group. Both types are characterized by frequent stools containing blood, mucus, and sometimes pus, with severe cramps and fever.

Dyspepsia. Simple indigestion, usually associated with excess stomach acidity; can become chronic if ignored.

Enteritis. Inflammation of any part of the intestine, caused by any one of several things: an abscess, a generalized inflammation, an obstruction, or malnutrition.

Food poisoning. Sometimes called ptomaine poisoning. There are bacterial poisonings such as botulism, nonbacterial such as that caused by eating toadstools (mistaking them for mushrooms), and poisoning caused by eating egg/fish/milk/poultry dishes which have stood without refrigeration for too long, thus developing cultures of harmful bacteria.

Gastritis. An acute inflammation of the stomach, sometimes severe in onset but usually of short duration. This may be caused by too much alcohol, highly spiced foods, or by bacteria such as streptococcus. A mild diet, an antacid, and one of the antispasmodic medications are the best regimen for relief.

Hemorrhoids. A swollen, inflamed portion of the rectum and/or anus, involving either or both the internal and external tissues, sometimes thrombosed (containing a clot). Surgery can be performed to remove the thrombosed area if it is severe enough. Bed rest and hemorrhoidal suppositories usually effect a cure.

Peptic ulcer. (also called a gastric ulcer) An erosion of the mucous membrane of the stomach or duodenum, caused by excessive secretion of acid gastric juice. Emotional and psychological problems play an important role in peptic ulcer. This type of ulcer is rarely larger than a quarter if in the stomach, or a dime if in the duodenum. Ulcers are three to four times more common in men than women. If the ulcer perforates, surgery usually must be performed.

Peritonitis. Inflammation of the peritoneum, the membrane lining the abdominal cavity. It can be caused by inflammation of the gastrointestinal tract, by inflammation of the female genital tract, by any penetration of the abdominal wall such as a stab wound, by bacteria such as streptococci, or by accidental "soiling" during surgery.

Pyloric tumor. Any tumor, malignant or benign, of the sphincter muscle at the lower end of the stomach. Sometimes these tumors become large enough to completely close the pylorus.

Rectal polyps. Small balloonlike growths or "bubbles" which grow along the walls of the rectum and sigmoid colon. If not removed (by simple surgery), they may cause cancer in that area.

Diseases of the Liver

Cirrhosis. A progressive chronic destruction of liver tissue, which can be caused by alcoholism, storage of bile in the liver, or toxic hepatitis. It may be triggered by nutritional deficiency, by infection, or by other as yet unknown factors. The liver becomes hardened and covered by hobnail deposits of fatty tissue.

Hepatitis. There are three types: viral hepatitis, infectious hepatitis, and toxic hepatitis. Viral hepatitis is one of the most common diseases in the United States. Hepatitis can be transmitted by mouth, by drinking water that is polluted, by swimming in dirty pools or lakes, or sometimes by blood transfusion. Pooled blood or plasma may contain the hepatitis virus, unknown and unrecognized by the doctor or pathologist. The virus is not killed by a 70% alcohol, but when stored at room temperature for over 6 months, appears to be safe; this of course applies only to plasma, not whole blood. All forms of hepatitis are accompanied by fever, nausea, loss of appetite and weight, and sometimes jaundice.

Jaundice. This is more properly a symptom than a disease. The skin becomes yellow, sometimes even orange or light green. Jaundice is caused by bile pigment in the blood. It may be caused by hepatitis, cirrhosis, cancer, liver failure, or by inhalation of carbon tetrachloride fumes.

Tumors and cancers of the liver are rare, but they do occur.

Diseases of the Spleen

Gaucher's disease. A rare disease causing enlargement of the spleen and jaundice. The bones soften, which seems to uphold the theory that the spleen controls the blood-building function of the bone marrow.

Hypercholesterolemic splenomegaly. Characterized by excessive fat cells in the blood (hyper/cholesterol/emic), obstruction of the bile duct, chronic pancreatitis, and an enlarged spleen.

Letterer-Siew disease. This disease affects young children, and runs a rapid and fatal course with enlargement of the spleen, anemia, and a skin eruption. Most body organs are damaged.

Niemann-Pick disease. Characterized by softening of the skull. Excessive fat cells show up in the adrenals, intestines, lungs, and brain.

Schüller-Christian disease. There is an excess of cholesterol, onset of diabetes insipidus, and softening of the skull. The pituitary gland is affected, and growth is stopped in children.

Splenomegaly. Enlargement of the spleen — sometimes it becomes twice its normal size and has been known to completely fill the abdominal cavity, probably due to its becoming engorged with blood.

Diseases of the Pancreas

Diabetes is the principal disease associated with the pancreas. There are two types: *growth-onset,* labile, or brittle diabetes, which occurs before skeletal growth is completed, and *maturity-onset,* occurring later in life, usually after age 40, known as diabetes mellitus. Diabetes insipidus is not a disease of the pancreas, but a disorder of the pituitary gland.

If the pancreas produces any insulin at all, diabetes can often be controlled by diet and oral antidiabetic medication. If the organ has ceased to produce any insulin, then insulin must be given by injection, daily. Dr. Frederick Banting, a Canadian physician, discovered in 1922 that insulin could be extracted from the pancreatic islets of animals. Until that time diabetes was a fatal disease.

Diabetes is definitely hereditary. It is wise to know if any of your family have it or have had it, and what their relation is to you. If both parents have diabetes, your chances of being diabetic are 100%. If one parent and an aunt or uncle on the other side of the family have diabetes, your chances are 85%. If one parent and a first cousin on the other side of the family have it, your chances are 40 to 60%. If one parent has diabetes and no one on the other side of the family is diabetic, your chances are still 22%. If you fit into any of these categories, you should have your doctor take a blood sugar test or a glucose tolerance test. The earlier the disease is detected, the better the chances for living a long, healthy life.

Pancreatitis (inflammation of the pancreas) is the second most common disease of the organ. The walls and arteries of the pancreas break down, the pancreatic duct is obstructed, and intense pain follows. Gallstones can bring on pancreatitis, as can alcoholism.

Cystic fibrosis is a pancreatic disease characterized by hardening of pancreatic tissue. Many cysts appear in the organ, and it becomes thick and fibrous. The liver is affected, and then the lungs. Death occurs from cirrhosis of the liver, pneumonia, or some other form of respiratory failure. Children are more often affected than adults.

Tumors and cancers of the pancreas are relatively common. Thrombosis results, causing numerous clots. The patient usually first shows signs of insulin coma, followed by convulsions. Recovery from convulsions can be rapid when large amounts of sugar are given. The only cure of tumor or cancer is removal of the organ.

TERMINOLOGY

Roots	Terms	Descriptions
bucca— cheek	bucco/lingual bucco/gingiv/itis	pertaining to the cheek and tongue inflammation of cheek and gums
chole— bile	chole/cyst chole/lith/otomy	the gallbladder incision to remove gallstones
col— colon	col/itis colon/algia	inflammation of the colon pain in the colon
enter— intestine	entero/cele entero/megaly	hernia, part of the intestine enlarged, dilated intestine
gastro— stomach	gastro/ptosis gastr/ostomy	dropping down of stomach more/less permanent opening, stomach
gingiva— gums	gingiv/itis gingivo/plasty	inflammation of the gums plastic surgery on the gums
hepato— liver	hepato/malacia hepato/pexy	softening of the liver surgical fixation of the liver

Roots	Terms	Descriptions
ile— *	ileo/necrosis	death of tissue, 3rd part small intestine
ileum	ileo/rrhaphy	suturing of intestinal tissue, ileum
lapar—	lapar/otomy	exploratory incision in abdomen
abdomen	laparo/myos/itis	inflammation of abdominal muscles
odont—	orth/odont/ist	dentist who straightens teeth
tooth	odont/algia	toothache
procto—	procto/scopy	inspection of rectum by instrument
rectum	proct/ology	study of rectal diseases
sial—	sial/aden/itis	inflammation of a salivary gland
saliva	sialo/lith	stone in a salivary gland
splen—	spleno/megaly	enlargement of the spleen
spleen	spleno/rrhexis	rupture of the spleen
viscer—	inter/visceral	occurring between two organs
organ	viscer/atonic	lack of normal tone in an organ

*NOTE: There are two roots which are almost identical: *ile,* the third part of the small intestine, the ileum, and *ili,* the hip bone or ilium. If you will remember that the root which ends in "e" matches with *enter,* or intestine, and the root which ends in "i" matches with *hip,* this may help to keep them straight in your mind.

You have also learned the following suffixes, as well as three additional roots and two prefixes:

aden—	gland (root)	*myo—*	muscle (root)
—algia	pain	*—necrosis*	death of tissue
—atonic	lack of tone	*—ology*	the study of
—cele	hernia	*ortho—*	straight (prefix)
—cyst	bladder, sac (root)	*—pexy*	surgical fixation of tissue
inter—	between (prefix)		
—malacia	softening	*—ptosis*	dropping downward
—megaly	enlargement	*—scopy*	inspection

Additional Vocabulary

absorb: to take up, as a blotter absorbs water (see also adsorb)

achlorhydria: absence of hydrochloric acid in gastric juices

acidosis: excess acid in the blood

adrenal corticoid: hormone manufactured by the outer cortex or covering of the adrenal glands

adsorb: to adhere to the surface, as sand to a sticky surface

albumin: a water-soluble protein, coagulable by heat (egg white contains a large percentage of albumin)

anacid: without acid, neutral, or alkaline

anorexia: lack or loss of appetite

antacid: medication to neutralize acid

bariatrics: the study of diet for weight reduction

emetic: medication or substance to induce vomiting

enzyme: organic substance produced in cells which causes change by catalytic action, as pepsin, a digestive enzyme

excrete: to throw off, as waste material, fecal matter

fibrinogen: protein in blood which forms network of a clot

G-I: abbreviation for gastrointestinal, as in G-I disease

glucose: sugar made by hydrolysis (breakdown) of carbohydrates

glycogen: animal starch (carbohydrate) stored in the liver

hormone: a chemical secreted into body fluid by an endocrine gland which has a specific effect on other organs of the body

metabolism: process by which food is turned into energy for body

necrosis: death or decay of tissue or bone

peristalsis: process of moving food along the digestive tract

pigment: coloring matter in cells and tissues

plasma: fluid part of blood in which corpuscles are suspended

prothrombin: forerunner of thrombin, which aids blood clotting

symptom: any manifestation of a disease or condition

syndrome: a set of symptoms

synthesis: a building and uniting of parts to make a whole unit

Pronunciations and Accents for Terms

acetone	ass'-eh-tone
achlorhydria	ay-klor-high'-dree-uh
adrenal	add-ree'-nal
amebae	am-ee'-bye
amino (acid)	am-ee'-no
anorexia	an-oh-rex'-ee-uh
anus	ay'-nus
bariatrics	bear-ee-at'-tricks
buccolingual	buck-oh-ling'-wall
buccopharyngeal	buck-oh-fair-in-jee'-al
cardia	kar'-dee-uh
cholecyst	coal'-ee-sist
cholecystectomy	coal-ee-sis-tek'-toe-me
cholecystitis	coal-ee-sis-tie'-tus
cholelithiasis	coal-ee-lith-eye'-ah-sis
cholelithotomy	coal-ee-lith-ott'-oh-me
chyme	kime (like time)
cirrhosis	sear-oh'-sis
colitis	coal-eye'-tis
colonalgia	coal-un-al'-jee-uh
colostomy	coal-oss'-toe-me
corticosteroid	kor-ti-ko-steer'-oyd
diabetes	die-uh-beet'-eez
insipidus	in-sip'-eh-dus
diabetes	die-uh-beet'-eez
mellitus	mell-eye'-tus
diverticulitis	die-ver-tik-you-lie'-tis
duodenum	dew-oh-dee'-num
emetic	ee-met'-ik
enterocolitis	en-ter-oh-coal-eye'-tis
enzyme	en'-zyme
epiglottis	ep-eh-glot'-tis
esophagus	ess-off'-ah-gus
excrete	ex-kreet'
fecal	fee'-kal
feces	fee'-sees
fibrinogen	fie-brin'-oh-jen
gastroptosis	gas-trop-toe'-sis

gastrotomy	gas-trot'-oh-me
gingivitis	jin-ji-vye'-tus
gingivolingual	jin-ji-voe-ling'-wall
glucose	glue'-kose
glycogen	gly'-ko-jen
hemorrhoid	hem'-or-oyd
hepatitis	hep-ah-tight'-iss
hepatolysis	hep-ah-tol'-ah-sis
hepatomegaly	hep-ah-toe-meg'-aly
ileostomy	ill-ee-oss'-toe-me
ileum	ill'-ee-um
intervisceral	in-ter-viss'-er-al
ketone	key'-tone
laparomegaly	lap-are-oh-meg'-ully
laparomyositis	lap-are-oh-my-oh-sigh'-tis
laparotomy	lap-are-ott'-oh-me
metabolism	met-tab'-oh-lizm
mucus	mew'-kuss
necrosis	nee-kro'-sis
odontalgia	oh-don-tal'-jee-uh
orthodontist	or-tho-don'-tist
pancreas	pan'-kree-us
peristalsis	pear-eh-stal'-sis
polyp	poll'-up
proctology	prok-tol'-uh-jee
proctoscopy	prok-tos'-ko-pee
prothrombin	pro-throm'-bin
ptyalin	tie'-uh-lin
pylorus	pie-loar'-us
salivary	sal'-eh-vary
sialadenitis	sigh-al-add-en-eye'-tis
sialolith	sigh-al'-oh-lith
sphincter	sfink'-ter
splenomegaly	splen-oh-meg'ully
syndrome	sin'-drome
synthesis	sin'-the-sis
thrombosis	throm-bow'-sis
villi	vil'-lee
viscera	viss'-er-ah

REVIEW TEST: THE DIGESTIVE AND EXCRETORY SYSTEMS

1. Name five parts of the digestive system.

2. Name three parts of the excretory system.

3. Name five diseases of the digestive system.

4. Define peristalsis.

5. Define pylorus.

6. Define hepatolysis.

7. Define cholecystectomy.

8. Define proctoscopy.

9. Define laparomyositis.

10. Define ileonecrosis.

11. Define gastroptosis.

12. Differentiate between gastrotomy and gastrostomy.

13. Differentiate between colitis and cholecystitis.

14. Explain cardiaspasm.

15. Give term for enlarged liver.

16. Give term for gallstones.

17. Give term for intestinal hernia.

18. Give term for pain in colon.

19. Give term for stone in salivary gland.

20. Define buccogingivitis.

3

THE SKELETAL AND MUSCULAR SYSTEMS

While the skeleton and muscles of the body are two separate "systems" they must be studied together because they work together: the skeleton supports the body and the muscles move it.

THE SKELETAL SYSTEM

How did we get the skeletal structure we now have? Radioactive potassium has given us a kind of atomic clock which tells us when man began to emerge — about 20 million years ago, when the earth's climate began to change. Heavy rains stopped, and grasslands began to develop. The trees provided food and shelter, but as population grew, prehistoric man had to move from the trees to the ground.

Our ancestors who left the trees were under 5 feet tall, weighed less than 90 pounds, and originally walked on all fours. Food had to be eaten on the ground and had therefore to be carried to a safe place for consumption. Man began to use his "front feet" or arms to lug food. Upright posture slowly began to develop. The spine had to begin to curve to carry the body upright. Hip sockets were changed to support weight. The buttock muscles grew larger and stronger to help hold the spine upright. Collarbones and clavicles altered to give arms more lifting strength. Biceps grew longer and stronger, legs lengthened, and feet enlarged and flattened. The foot developed an arch to act as a shock absorber for body weight in walking and running. Jaws which had moved up and down developed a rolling motion to chew meat. The new chewing motion developed a jutting jaw, changing the shape of the face. Because man had to grow shrewd to survive, his brain developed too.

In standing erect, man found he could see over the high grass, giving him an advantage over his enemies.

The Spine

To man as an upright animal, the spinal column is extremely important and merits a brief separate discussion. In creatures who travel on all fours, the spine is like a bridge or a clothesline with all the organs hanging vertically from the vertebrae. For man, walking on two feet, the spine becomes an upright column which must not only support the body weight, but be able to twist, bend, and move at any angle.

The spine houses the spinal cord, a cable along which 31 pairs of nerves are strung. About half of these are *sensory* nerves which carry messages *to* the brain, while the rest are *motor* nerves used to carry information *from* the brain to muscles.

There are 33 bones, or *vertebrae*, in the spine. The 7 cervical vertebrae allow us to look up, down, around, and twist our necks. The 12 thoracic vertebrae are more restricted in movement and serve to protect the heart, lungs, and chest. The 5 lumbar vertebrae carry most of our weight and are most likely to suffer from abuse. Below the lumbar vertebrae are the 5 fused sacral vertebrae, and below these are the 4 fused vertebrae which form the coccyx, or tail bone.

Between each pair of vertebrae there is a cushion called a *disc*, made up of cartilage and containing a gelatinous substance. If a disc is damaged in a fall or other injury, it may press on a nerve and cause a muscle to go into spasm. A ruptured disc often presses on the sciatic nerve, which runs down the leg and causes pain to radiate to the leg and foot.

There are 400 muscles and 1000 ligaments in the support system of the human spine. The amount of proper exercise we get and the posture we maintain, both sitting and standing, are largely responsible for a "good" or a "bad" back. The use of a firm mattress and firm, straight chairs are a great help for a healthy back. Exercise in the form of walking, provided proper posture is maintained, is also helpful. The way we pick things up and lift them has an effect on the back, as well. We should always squat when lifting, bending the knees and keeping the spine straight.

To avoid pain, injury, and discomfort with advancing age, it is wise to check your posture: Bending the knees very slightly and with the feet slightly apart, back up to a wall. Perfect posture would make it possible for the entire spinal area to touch the wall. Slip your hand behind the "small of the back," and if there is space there, make an effort to push that area of the back in to the wall. Checking posture frequently and keeping the back as straight as possible decreases back trouble.

The Skeleton

The skeleton has three functions: (1) provides locomotion of the body; (2) supports the tissues and muscles; and (3) protects the body by giving it structural support. The skeleton is divided into three main parts: the skull, the trunk, and the extremities. Picture the skeleton as similar to the steel framework which holds up a building.

A bone is made up of a head, a shaft, a tough covering, and an inner marrow. The *head* is the rounded end of the bone where it meets another bone or fastens into a socket. The *shaft* is the main part of the bone, its length. The *marrow* is the central inner core of the bone which contains blood vessels to nourish the bone cells. Red blood cells are manufactured in the bone marrow. This process is called *hematopoiesis*.

There are five types of bones:

1. **Flat** — clavicle, pelvis, sacrum, ribs, sternum
2. **Short** — carpals, metacarpals, tarsals, metatarsals
3. **Long** — humerus, femur, tibia, fibula, radius, ulna
4. **Hinge-joint** — ankle, elbow, jaw, knee, wrist
5. **Ball-and-socket** — hip, shoulder

Compare the following numbered parts of the skeleton with the corresponding numbers in Fig. 3.

1. The **skull**, or bones of the head, which is made up of 7 parts. (see the insert in Fig. 3.)
2. **Cervical vertebrae**, the first 7 bones of the spine in the neck area.
3. **Thoracic vertebrae**, the next 12 bones of the spine in the chest area.
4. **Lumbar vertebrae**, the last 5 bones of the spine in the lower back.
5. **Sacrum**, the wide bone at the end of the spine which joins the two pelvic bones to make up the pelvic girdle.
6. **Coccyx**, the "tail bone" at the tip end of the spine.
7. **Clavicle**, the "collar bone," joined to the sternum in front and the scapula in back.
8. **Scapula**, the "shoulder blade," which protects the lungs at the back of the body and serves as an attachment for muscles of the arm.
9. **Humerus**, the long bone in the upper arm from shoulder to elbow.

10. **Radius**, the smaller bone in the lower arm from elbow to wrist, works with the humerus and ulna at the elbow. This bone is on the side of the arm toward the thumb.
11. **Ulna**, the larger bone of the lower arm, on the side of the arm toward the little finger.
12. **Sternum**, the flat bone running from the joining of the clavicles to the end of the ribs, in the front of the body.
13. **Carpals**, the 8 bones of the wrist which make it flexible.
14. **Metacarpals**, the 5 bones of the palms of the hand.
15. **Phalanges**, the 14 small finger bones, 3 in each finger, 2 in the thumb.
16. **Ilium**, the large flat hip bone which helps to form the pelvic bowl.
17. **Femur**, the long thigh bone which fits into a ball-and-socket joint at the hip.
18. **Patella**, the round bone covering the knee joint (the "kneecap").
19. **Ribs**, of which there are 12 pairs. Ten pairs attach to the sternum; the last 2 pairs are called "floating" ribs because they are attached only to the vertebrae.
20. **Tibia**, the larger leg bone joining the femur and fibula, on the side of the leg toward the big toe.
21. **Fibula**, the smaller leg bone joining the femur, on the side of the little toe.
22. **Tarsals**, the 7 bones of the ankle which give movement to the foot.
23. **Metatarsals**, the 5 bones of the instep.
24. **Phalanges**, the 14 small toe bones corresponding to the phalanges in the fingers.
25. **Calcaneus**, the round heel bone (one of the tarsal bones).

DISEASES AND DISORDERS

Skeletal Diseases

Arthritis. Inflammation of the joints, usually with pain, often resulting in deformities of hands, feet, and knees as the disease advances.

Bursitis. Inflammation of a bursa (a sac filled with fluid that allows a joint to move easily), causing extreme pain when the joint is moved.

Calcifications. Calcium deposits on or around any bone, causing pain or discomfort on movement.

Gout. The result of an abnormal amount of uric acid in the system, usually starting with involvement of the big toe. Alcohol and large amounts of protein aggravate the disease.

THE SKELETON (Rear view)

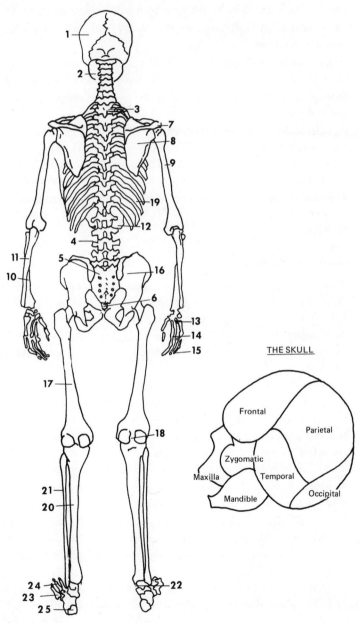

THE SKULL

Figure 3

49

Osteoarthritis. A chronic, degenerative joint disease, usually seen in elderly people. The joints thicken and cause pain when movement is made.

Osteomalacia. A softening of the bones with pain, tenderness, and muscular weakness.

Osteomyelitis. Inflammation and infection of the bones caused by bacteria, which may spread through the bone and cause pus to form.

Osteoporosis. A porous condition of the bones, making them more brittle and easily broken.

Poliomyelitis. An acute disease characterized by high fever, sore throat, and involvement of the central nervous system and the spine, often ending in paralysis of parts of the body. The disease is now almost completely eliminated through the use of Salk vaccine and other polio vaccines.

Tuberculosis of the bone. A form of tuberculosis originating in the bones, causing degeneration and decay. It is now treated successfully with antibiotics.

Skeletal Malformations

Achondroplasia. The dwarf, usually under 4 feet tall with a large head, short arms and legs. These people are sometimes of subnormal intelligence. The disease is due to improper development of cartilage during childhood.

Acromegaly. Characterized by a large head, huge hands and feet, a lantern jaw, and spinal deformities. The disease is due to excessive pituitary secretion.

Giantism. These people sometimes reach a height of 8 feet or more due to an excess of growth hormones. There is no treatment or known cure. Patients usually die young, in their twenties.

Hip dislocation. Fairly common in newborn babies. Dislocation can be corrected during the first year of life by surgery or the application of a kind of orthopedic spreading harness, to straighten hip joints.

Kyphosis. Commonly called hunchback, this is an exaggerated outward curve of the thoracic portion of the spine.

Lipochondystrophy (gargoylism). Characterized by a short stubby trunk, curved spine, enlarged liver and spleen, deformed nose, and jutting lower jaw. These people are usually emotionally unstable, and die young.

Midget. This is the hypopituitary "doll" from 24 to 36 inches tall, perfectly proportioned, intelligent, and able to produce normal children. The disease is due to a deficiency of growth hormones. When it is discovered and corrected with hormonal treatment in infancy, these people can grow to normal size, while dwarfs cannot.

Osteogenesis imperfecta (brittle bones). Patients have almost constant fractures, usually are cripples before age 20, and often deaf at an early age. The only treatment is to try to protect them from falls and bumps.

Rickets. A vitamin-deficiency disease due to lack of vitamin D, calcium, and sunshine. The bones are distorted, as in bowlegs.

Scoliosis. Commonly called curvature of the spine. The vertebral column is curved out of normal alignment, usually sideways.

Scurvy. A vitamin-deficiency disease due to lack of vitamin C, fresh fruits, vegetables, and milk; characterized by weakness and anemia.

THE MUSCULAR SYSTEM

Motion of the body is made possible by coordination of the skeletal and muscular systems. Muscles initiate movement of the body from place to place, bending, stretching, breathing, the beating of the heart, smiling, frowning, speaking, and the movements of the digestive and circulatory systems.

There are four types of muscles:

1. **Skeletal.** These are voluntary muscles, enabling body movements, facial expressions, etc.
2. **Visceral.** These are involuntary muscles found in the walls of body organs, including blood vessels. The smooth muscles in blood vessels produce changes in size as needed by the body in activity. The muscles of the digestive tract and those of the bladder, kidneys, etc., belong in this class.
3. **Cardiac.** These muscles maintain the action of the heart. The rhythm of heartbeat is controlled by a network of cardiac muscles over which impulses pass in every direction. These are also involuntary muscles.
4. **Sphincter.** These muscles are round and move as if threaded with elastic, opening and closing. Voluntary sphincter muscles are located in the bladder, esophagus, urethra, rectum, and anus. Involuntary sphincter muscles are those of the cardia, bile duct, pylorus, prostate, ovaries, fallopian tubes, veins, and arteries.

Tendons are fibrous cords by which a muscle is attached to a bone. **Ligaments** are bands of connective tissue which connect adjacent bones to muscles, or which help to support body organs. Tendons are cords; ligaments are bands.

DISEASES AND DISORDERS

Cerebral palsy. Caused by damage to the motor nerves, usually the result of a birth injury. These patients are "spastics." Sometimes they walk normally when the Achilles tendon (at the back of the heel) is cut, since this tendon partially controls our gait and manner of walking.

Charleyhorse. Simple soreness and stiffness in a muscle, caused by strain. It is a temporary condition, relieved by heat and massage.

Chorea (St. Vitus Dance). A convulsive nervous disease causing involuntary jerking movements of the body. Chorea can be hereditary. There are 54 types of chorea.

Multiple sclerosis. This disease causes double vision, temporary blindness, and general aches and pains. Portions of the brain and the spine harden; nervous reflexes weaken and stop. Patients have little control over the muscles.

Muscular cramps and spasm. Usually caused by strain, sprain, or being overly tired, but may be caused by the lack of some vitamin. This is a temporary condition, not a disease.

Muscular dystrophy. A progressive weakening of the muscles, cause unknown. Patients usually end up in wheel chairs when muscles become uncontrollable.

Myasthenia gravis. A disease involving the involuntary muscles, which may be caused by a diseased thymus gland. Patients have difficulty speaking and usually die of a respiratory infection.

Myositis. Inflammation of any voluntary muscle.

Palsy. There are many types of palsy, all of which cause the head, hands, and lips to quiver and shake, and otherwise affect muscular activity.

Pulled or torn ligaments. Caused by strain, sprain, and accident, or overly strenuous activity; common in football players and wrestlers.

Talipes. A deformity affecting both the bones and muscles. Commonly called "club foot," this deformity twists the foot out of proper position. It can be corrected very shortly after birth with simple surgery.

Tendinitis. Inflammation of a tendon or a muscle-tendon attachment; common in tennis players.

Tenosynovitis. Inflammation of the sheath or covering of a tendon.

TERMINOLOGY APPLICABLE TO THE SKELETAL AND MUSCULAR SYSTEMS

Roots	Terms	Descriptions
arthro— joint	arthr/itis arthro/desis	inflammation of a joint surgical fixation of joint
caud— tail (coccyx)	caudio/cephalad caudio/spinal	from tail to head pertaining to coccyx & spine
cephalo— head	cephal/algia cephalo/centesis	pain in the head; headache surgical puncture of head
cerebro— brain	cerebro/sarcoma cerebr/otomy	cancer of the brain incision into the brain
chondro— cartilage	chondr/oma costo/chondral	a cartilaginous tumor pertaining to ribs & cartilage
cranio— skull (cranium)	cranio/malacia cranio/sclerosis	softening of bones of skull hardening of skull bones
dactyl— finger, toe	dactyl/edema dactylo/megaly	excess fluid in fingers, toes enlarged fingers, toes
fascia— band (tissue)	fascia/plasty fascio/rrhaphy	plastic surgery on fascia suturing any fascia tissue
ili— ilium (hip bone)	ili/ectomy ilio/sacral	surgical removal of hip bone pertaining to ilium & sacrum
mening— membrane	mening/eal mening/itis	relating to a membrane inflammation of membrane around the brain and spinal cord
myelo— marrow (bone)	myelo/cyte myelo/fibr/osis	any bone marrow cell fibrous tissue replacing bone marrow
myo— muscle	myo/cardium myo/cele	the muscle(s) of the heart hernia of any muscle
osteo— bone	osteo/myel/itis osteo/porosis	disease of bone & marrow porous condition of a bone

(continued)

Roots	Terms	Descriptions
ped—,	ped/arthr/itis	arthritis of the foot
pod— foot	pod/iatrics	study of foot disorders
spondyl— spine, vertebrae	spondylo/plegia spondylo/syn/desis	paralysis of the spine fixation of vertebrae

We have added the following suffixes to our vocabulary:

—cyte	cell (root)	*—sclerosis*	hardening, thickening
—desis	surgical fixation of bone or joint (*—pexy* for tissue)	*—syndesis*	surgical fixation of vertebrae; only place in the body where two or more bones are aligned in continuous process.
—edema	swelling due to excess fluid		
—iatric	study or practice of		
—plegia	paralysis		
—porosis	porous condition		

Additional Vocabulary

abductor: *ab*=away, *duct*=pull. Abductor muscles pull away from the body.

adductor: *ad*=toward. Adductor muscles pull toward the body.

afferent: toward, or to convey toward the center (see efferent)

anterior: toward the front or front part of body (see posterior)

atrophy: to shrivel or shrink, as in muscular atrophy

CVA: cerebrovascular accident; a stroke — included here because a stroke usually affects the muscles

distal: away from, as the dorsolumbar region of the spine

dystrophy: in this case, *dys* means faulty, though usually it means painful or difficult; *trophia*=nourish; together, they mean faulty nourishment, sometimes of bones or muscles.

efferent: away from, pushing out from the center

epiphysis: portions of bone separated in early life by cartilage, which with maturity grow together; where cartilage exists in an infant, this is the epiphysis; bones can lengthen here as the body grows.

extension: straightening out after flexion (see flexion)

fascia: a band of fibrous tissue which aids the muscles in movement, as in abdominal fascia

flexion: bending, as in flexing an arm or leg

ganglion: a mass of nerve cells which form a knot on a joint or tumor on a tendon

i.m.: intramuscular; injection into the muscle

inferior: toward the bottom (see superior)

intermediate: between, or in the middle

medial: toward the middle

orthopedic: the study of the skeletal structure or referring to it

posterior: toward the back, or rear of the body

proximal: near the source, nearest any point being described

striated: striped, or in bands, as in muscular bands

superficial: near the surface

superior: toward the top, or above

trephine: the process of removing a circular piece of bone from the skull for examination, used frequently in brain surgery

Pronunciations and Accents for Terms

Achilles	Ah-kill′-eez
achondroplasia	aye-kon-dro-play′-zee-uh
acromegaly	ak-row-meg′-ally
alimentary	al-eh-men′-tear-ee
arthrodesis	ar-throw-dee′-sis
calcaneus	kal-kain-′ee-us
carpal	kar′-pal
caudiocephalad	kaw-dee-oh-sef′-ah-lad
caudiospinal	kaw-dee-oh-spy′-nal
cephalalgia	sef-al-al′-gee-uh
cephalocentesis	sef-al-oh-sen-tee′-sis
cerebrosarcoma	sear-ee-bro-sar-ko′-ma
cerebrotomy	sear-ee-brot′-oh-me
chondroma	kon-dro′-ma

(continued)

Pronunciations and Accents for Terms (continued)

chorea	kore-ee'uh
clavicle	clav'-eh-kul
coccyx	kok'-six
costochondral	cost-oh-kon'-dral
craniomalacia	crane-ee-oh-mal-aye'-sha
craniomegaly	crane-ee-oh-meg'-ully
cranioisclerosis	crane-ee-oh-skler-oh'-sis
dactyledema	dak-till-eh-dee-'ma
dactylomegaly	dak-till-oh-meg'-ully
dystrophy	dis'-tro-fee
endocrine	en'-do-krin
epiphysis	ee-pif'-eh-sis
fallopian	fal-low'-pe-un
fasciaplasty	fash'-ee-uh-plas-tee
fasciorrhaphy	fash-ee-oh'-raf-ee
femur	fee'-mer
fibula	fib'-you-la
ganglion	gang'-glee-un
hematopoiesis	heem-at-oh-poy-ee'-sus
humerus	hew'-mer-us
iliectomy	ill-ee-ek'-toe-me
iliosacral	ill-ee-oh-sake'-rall
ilium	ill'-ee-um
kyphosis	ky-fo'-sis
lipochondystrophy	lip-oh-kon-diss'-tro-fee
mandible	man'-dib-ul
maxilla	max'-ill-uh
medial	meed'-ee-ul
meningeal	men-in-gee'-al
meningioma	men-in-jee-oh'-ma
meningitis	men-in-jy'-tis
metacarpal	met-ah-kar'-pal
metatarsal	met-ah-tar'-sal
myasthenia	my-as-thee'-ne-uh
myelitis	my-el-eye'-tis
myelocyte	my'-el-oh-sight
myelofibrosis	my-el-oh-fy-bro'-sis
myelosarcoma	my-el-oh-sar-ko'-ma

myocardium	my-oh-kar'-de-um
myocarditis	my-oh-kar-die'-tis
myocele	my'-oh-seal
myositis	my-oh-sigh'-tis
occipital	ok-sip'-eh-tal
osteoarthritis	oss-tee-oh-ar-thry'-tis
osteogenesis	os-tee-oh-jen'-eh-sis
osteomalacia	os-tee-oh-may-lay'-she-uh
osteomyelitis	os-tee-oh-my-el-eye'-tis
osteoporosis	os-tee-oh-pore-oh'-sis
parietal	pair-eye'-eh-tal
patella	pa-tell'-ah
pedarthritis	ped-ar-thry'-tis
pelvis	pell'-viss
phalanges	fay-lan'-jeez
pituitary	pi-chew'-eh-tary
podiatrics	po-dee-at'-tricks
poliomyelitis	po-lee-oh-my-eh-lie'-tis
prostate	pros'-tate
sacrum	sake'-rum
scapula	skap'-yew-la
sclerosis	skler-oh'-sis
scoliosis	sko-lee-oh'-sis
scurvy	skur'-vee
spondylolisthesis	spon-dil-oh-lis-thee'-sis
spondylosyndesis	spon-dil-oh-sin-dee'-sis
sternum	ster'-num
striate	stree'-ate
talipes	tal'-eh-peez
tarsal	tar'-sal
tendinitis	ten-din-eye'-tis
tenosynovitis	ten-oh-sigh-no-vy'-tis
thoracic	tho-rass'-ik
tibia	tib'-ee-uh
trephine	tree'-fine
ulna	ull'-na
vertebrae	ver'-te-bray
vertebral	ver-tee'-bral
zygomatic	zy-go-mat'-ik

REVIEW TEST: THE SKELETAL AND MUSCULAR SYSTEMS

1.   Name three parts of any bone.

2.   Name the five types of bones.

3.   Name the three spinal divisions.

4.   Name three joints in the body.

5.   Name the four types of muscles.

6.   Define osteomalacia.

7.   Define arthrodesis.

8.   Define craniosclerosis.

9.   Define dactylomegaly.

10. Define iliectomy.

11. Name three muscular diseases.

12. Name four skeletal diseases.

13. Differentiate between myelitis and myositis.

14. Differentiate between chondroma and cerebroma.

15. Define scoliosis.

16. Define kyphosis.

17. Give term for surgical puncture of the head.

18. Give term for hernia of a muscle.

19. Give term for tumor of a membrane.

20. Give term for headache.

4

THE CARDIOVASCULAR AND CIRCULATORY SYSTEMS

The heart, the chief organ of the cardiovascular system, can be pictured as a large muscle, for its major activity is muscular; it contracts and relaxes at an average rate of 75-85 times each minute. Each contraction takes 8/10 of a second. The relaxation period is about 1 second. The heart really is at rest longer than it is at work, but the whole heart doesn't rest all at one time; some parts rest while others are working.

The sounds we hear when listening to the heartbeat are made by the opening and closing of the valves. Each minute, 5 quarts of blood pass through the heart. Since we have 6-7 quarts of blood, almost the entire blood supply is cleaned and circulated every minute. Looking at Fig. 4, you can follow the route of the blood through the heart.

"Used" blood which has circulated through the body enters the heart through the *superior* and *inferior vena cava,* two large veins at the top and bottom of the heart area. This blood goes first to the *right atrium,* then down to the *right ventricle,* and up through the *pulmonary artery* to the lungs. Freshly oxygenated blood from the lungs enters the heart through the *pulmonary veins,* into the *left atrium,* down to the *left ventricle,* then up and out through the *aorta,* to circulate again through the body.

The circulatory system is a complex network of tubes. The network which carries the blood away from the heart consists of:

The *aorta,* which loops behind the heart and goes down back of the stomach until it branches to form the right and left common iliac arteries.

The *arteries,* made of an elasticized tissue. There are more than 300 principal arteries in the body.

The *arterioles,* smaller than the arteries, which branch off from the arteries and are a thinner tissue, numbering in the thousands.

The *capillaries,* which branch off from the arterioles. These are very tiny hairlike tubes connecting arterioles with venules, and are countless.

The network which carries the blood *back to the heart* consists of:

The *veins,* tubes similar to arteries. There are more than 600 principal veins in the body.

The *venules,* smaller vessels corresponding to and connected with arterioles. These also number in the thousands.

Blood contains proteins, salts, enzymes, oxygen, carbon dioxide, and 91% water content. Blood is made up of these cells:

Erythrocytes, red cells or corpuscles which carry oxygen and contain *hemoglobin.* There are about 6 million erythrocytes to 1 cc of blood, or 30 million to a teaspoonful.

Leukocytes, the white cells or corpuscles. These fight infection and are larger than erythrocytes; there are about 35,000 of these to a teaspoonful.

Lymphocytes, cells produced in the lymph glands, which help to regulate body processes and fight foreign matter in blood.

Monocytes, cells with a single nucleus, which carry protoplasm (a fluid which makes up the essential material of all plant and animal cells).

Macrocytes, large cells formed in the bone marrow.

Platelets, tiny cells concerned with blood coagulation.

The blood also contains *plasma,* the clear liquid in which the cells are suspended; *fibrinogen,* a factor in clotting and coagulation; and *prothrombin,* a second coagulation factor. *Antibodies,* carried in the plasma, are formed or synthesized when the body has been attacked by some disease (such as measles) and thereafter protect the body from repeated attacks; these are manufactured by lymphoid tissue and react against *antigens* to provide immunity.

Installation of a Pacemaker for the Heart

In 1960 three heart surgeons developed a small transistorized pacemaker to be installed permanently in the chest of patients suffering from heart blocks, which are often the result of a coronary occlusion. The pacemaker controls the rate of heartbeat and stimulates the heart to

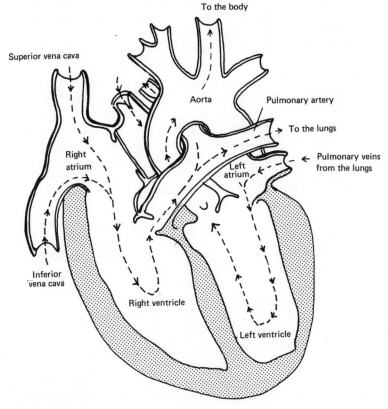

THE HEART

Figure 4

continue beating by using tiny electrodes implanted inside the heart muscle. The pacemaker can be set to the normal rate of the patient's own heart action by adjustment of the electrodes, which are connected to a very small object placed in the chest below the heart. Pacemakers have been shaped like a box, a ball, or a disc. Original pacemakers contained batteries and had to be replaced about every 5 years; now they can be operated by other methods, and will last a lifetime.

Deep anesthesia is necessary for this surgery, using hypothermia and a heart-lung pump-oxygenator as well. The anesthetic is generally administered, then a tube inserted into the trachea, with a small balloon at the lower end to enable the anesthetist to deflate and expand the lungs as necessary.

While the pacemaker is being installed, a large hospital pacemaker keeps the patient's heart beating at its normal rate. After the patient has been anesthetized, novocain is injected in the arm and the large vein at the inner bend of the elbow is opened (this is called a cut-down). A catheter is then placed in the cut-down, threaded up the arm, through the vena cava, pointed down toward the right atrium, and with the aid of a fluoroscope is put exactly in place inside the heart. At this point the large hospital pacemaker takes over the heart action. Now the patient is ready for the actual surgery.

This is the way the surgery progresses: An incision is made over the fourth rib, and the rib is removed. The pericardium (sac enclosing the heart) is opened and a small incision made in the heart muscle where the electrode will be placed. The electrode or electrodes are sutured to the heart muscle, then the muscle is sutured, and the pericardium is closed and sutured. The electrodes are connected to a small antenna coil attached to the miniature pacemaker, and this is placed just beneath the skin in the chest. Then the outer skin is sutured and the operation is over. The heart is automatically stimulated by radiowave impulses originating in the little pacemaker the patient now wears inside his chest. The fourth rib that was removed will eventually rebuild itself.

The wound is dressed and the patient sent to the recovery room. After 24 hours an electrocardiogram is taken to be sure the apparatus is performing as expected. On the second day the patient is walking around. All that remains to be done is to remove the stitches when the wound has healed.

This surgery has been performed hundreds of times in all parts of the world on patients ranging in age from a few weeks to the late eighties.

Each year improvements are made; in the years since the operation was originated it has become more reliable and permanent with each new version.

DISEASES AND DISORDERS

Cardiovascular Disorders

Chronic valvular heart disease. Permanent deformity of a heart valve which increases the heart's work load and leads to heart failure.

Congestive heart failure. Failure of the heart to provide an adequate blood supply to the tissues and organs of the body; occurs more frequently in older people.

Coronary arteriosclerosis. A progressive thickening of the inner lining of the coronary arteries, leading to clotting and obstruction.

Coronary atherosclerosis. Deposits of fatty cells or tissue in the coronary arteries; usually a disease of older people, more common in men than in women.

Coronary occlusion. A heart attack brought on by the closing of one of the coronary arteries, usually because of a clot.

Endocarditis. Inflammation of the membrane (endocardium) lining the cavities of the heart.

Myocarditis. Inflammation of one or more of the heart muscles, causing enlargement of the heart, and leading to congestive heart failure.

Paroxysmal tachycardia. A condition in which the pacemaker or regulator of the heart's rhythm temporarily functions abnormally, causing the heart to beat extremely rapidly — usually the result of fear, anxiety, or shock; not an organic disorder, but functional.

Pericarditis. Inflammation of the membrane covering the heart (the pericardium). Layers of fibrous tissue bind the layers of the pericardium.

Rheumatic heart disease. Occurs in rheumatic fever, causing inflammation of the endocardium, pericardium, and myocardium.

Congenital Heart Defects

Atrial septal defect. When a baby is born without a wall between the right and left atrium, blood flows directly from one to the other — can sometimes be corrected by surgery.

Patent ductus arteriosus. In the period before birth a baby gets his blood supply through a duct leading into the aorta. If this duct does not close at birth, the heart cannot work normally.

Pulmonary stenosis. The pulmonary artery and valve are obstructed, causing a "smothering" of the ventricle — can sometimes be corrected by surgery.

Operative Procedures

Cardiopulmonary bypass. Blood is diverted away from the heart by the use of a heart-lung pump-oxygenator to enable the surgeon to bypass the heart and lungs and work in a bloodless field.

Closed heart massage. Not a surgical procedure but one in which the physician rather violently compresses the heart by hand, in an effort to force blood into the aorta and begin heart action when the heart has stopped (cardiac arrest).

Open heart massage. The chest is opened and the heart is massaged manually in an effort to start the heart working again after a cardiac arrest.

Pericardiectomy. Incision and partial dissection of the pericardium to relieve the heart from adhesions caused by pericarditis.

Valvotomy. Repair of a heart valve by scraping, enlarging with a plastic tube, or rerouting the blood flow by attachment to another valve in better condition.

Circulatory Diseases or Malfunctions

Anemia. A deficiency of iron in the blood, or a deficiency of erythrocytes, or a deficiency in the quantity or quality of the blood, depending upon the type of anemia. There are over 100 types.

Angina pectoris. A block somewhere in the blood flow which causes the heart muscles to go into spasm. Severe chest pain is felt, also radiating down the left arm.

Aortic aneurysm. A major rupture in the aorta caused by a weak spot in the aortic wall. Immediate surgery may save the patient; sometimes an aortic transplant can be successfully accomplished.

Arteriosclerosis. Aside from coronary arteriosclerosis, the same thickening and eventual closure of arteries anywhere in the body may occur. Cerebral arteriosclerosis, for example, occurs in the arteries of the brain.

Blue baby. An infant born with an imperfect heart may have a lack of oxygen in the blood, creating cyanosis (a blue look to the skin). This can now be cured by surgery in most cases.

Coronary thrombosis. A blocking of blood flow to the heart, caused by a clot in any coronary artery.

Leukemia. A fatal disease of the blood-manufacturing processes — may be acute or chronic. There is a gradual but marked decrease in white blood cells, an enlarged spleen, and a breakdown of the lymph glands. Very new drugs can now bring about remissions (abatement of symptoms) but no cure has yet been found. There are many types.

Mononucleosis. An acute infectious disease characterized by sudden fever and swelling of the lymph nodes in the throat. An abnormal number of monocytes are found in the blood. Mononucleosis is also called "student's disease," because it usually attacks when the person is overtired and the body is "run down." Complete rest and a high-protein diet are necessary for recovery. Recurrences of the disease are frequent.

TERMINOLOGY

Roots	Terms	Descriptions
angio— *phleb—* vein, vessel	angio/cele phleb/itis	hernia of a blood vessel inflammation of a vein or veins
cardio— heart	cardio/genic cardio/pulmonary	originating within the heart involving heart and lungs
cyt— cell	cyto/penia erythro/cyt/osis	deficiency of any type cells disease of red blood cells
hemo— blood	hemo/stasis hemat/uria	stoppage of blood flow blood in the urine

Suffix	Terms	Description
—cyte cell	leuko/cyte mono/cyte	white blood cell single-nucleus cell
—penia deficiency	leuko/penia neutro/penia	deficiency of white blood cells deficiency of neutrophils in blood
—rrhagia hemorrhage	metro/rrhagia rhino/rrhagia	hemorrhage from the uterus hemorrhage from the nose

Suffix	Terms	Description
—stasis stoppage	cardio/stasis uro/stasis	heart stoppage stoppage of urine

Prefix	Terms	Description
brady— slow	brady/cardia	abnormally slow heartbeat
ecto— *exo—* outside	ecto/pic pregnancy exo/genous	pregnancy outside the uterus occurring outside the body
endo— inside, within	endo/genous endo/card/itis	occurring within the body inflammation inside the heart
hyper— excessive	hyper/tension hyper/glyc/emia	high blood pressure abnormal amount of sugar in blood or excessive blood sugar content
hypo— deficient	hypo/thyroid/ism hypo/glyc/emia	deficient thyroid gland activity below-normal blood sugar content
peri— around	peri/cardium peri/osteum	membrane surrounding the heart membrane covering the bones
tachy— rapid	tachy/cardia tachy/pnea tachy/phasia	abnormally rapid heartbeat abnormally rapid breathing extremely rapid speech

Additional Vocabulary

aneurysm: a weak spot in a vessel, vein, tube or artery which may rupture.

BMR: basal metabolism rate, the rate at which energy is used by the body.

BUN: blood urea nitrogen, a test for urea (part of the urine) in the blood

carotid: large artery on either side of the neck

CBC: complete blood count

congenital: existing at, and usually before, birth

coronary: corona = crown; the arteries encircling the heart

diastolic: blood pressure at the point of *dilation* of the heart (see systolic). If the systolic pressure is 120 and the diastolic is 90, it will be written as 120/90.

ecchymosis: free blood beneath the skin's surface, as in a blood blister

ECG/EKG: electrocardiogram, a tracing of heart activity

embolus: *a clot which has moved about,* obstructing circulation (see thrombus)

erythema: reddened skin due to a rash, flush, or inflammation

erythematosus: a form of lupus; lupus vulgaris is tuberculosis of the skin

ESR: erythrocyte sedimentation rate; a blood test

F.B.S.: fasting blood sugar; a test for diabetes

hyperemia: an excess of blood in any part of the body; not the same as ecchymosis

infarction: dead tissue caused by obstruction of a vessel

insult: used in medicine to denote injury, as a cardiac insult

I.V.: intravenous; injection into a vein

parenteral: not oral; intravenous, intramuscular, or injectable

RBC: red blood cell count

sphygmomanometer: the instrument used to measure blood pressure

systolic: blood pressure at the point of *contraction* of the heart (see diastolic)

thrombus: *a clot which remains where it is formed,* obstructing circulation

Pronunciations and Accents for Terms

anemia	ah-nee'-me-uh
aneurysm	an'-you-rizm
angiectomy	an-jee-ek'-to-me
angina pectoris	an-jy'-nah pek'-tore-us
angiocele	an'-jee-oh-seal
antigen	an'-teh-jen
aorta	ay-or'-ta
arteriole	ar-tear'-ee-ole
arteriosclerosis	ar-tear-ee-oh-skler-oh'-sis
atherosclerosis	ay-ther-oh-skler-oh'-sis

(continued)

Pronunciations and Accents for Terms (continued)

atrial septal defect	ay'-tree-al sep'-tal defect
atrium	ay'-tree-um
bradycardia	bray-dee-kar'-dee-uh
bradyphasia	bray-dee-fay'-zee-uh
capillary	kap'-eh-lary
cardiogenic	kar-dee-oh-jen'-ik
cardiopulmonary	kar-dee-oh-pull'-mon-ary
cardiostasis	kar-dee-oh-stay'-sis
cardiovascular	kar-dee-oh-vas'-kew-lar
carotid	kah-rot'-id
cholesterol	coal-ess'-ter-all
congenital	kon-jen'-eh-tal
cyanosis	sigh-ah-no'-sis
cyanotic	sigh-ah-not'-ik
cytolysis	sit-oll'-eh-sis
cytopenia	sit-oh-pee'-nee-uh
diastolic	die-uh-stol'-ik
ecchymosis	ek-kee-mo'-sis
ectocardial	ek-to-kar'-dee-ul
ectopic	ek-top'-ik
electrocardiogram	ee-lek-tro-kar'-dee-oh-gram
embolus	em'-bo-lus
endocarditis	en-do-kar-die'-tis
endogenous	en-doj'-en-us
eosinophil	ee-oh-sin'-oh-fill
erythema	err-eh-thee'-ma
erythematosus	err-eh-thee-ma-to'-sus
erythrocyte	ee-rith'-ro-site
erythrocytosis	ee-rith-ro-sit-oh'-sis
exogenous	ex-oj'-en-us
fibrinogen	fie-brin'-oh-jen
hematuria	heem-ah-tew'-ree-uh
hemoglobin	hee'-mo-glow-bin
hemolytic	he-mo-lit'-ik
hemostasis	he-mo-stay'-sis
hypercholesterolemic	hy-per-kol-ess-ter-ol-ee'-mik
hyperemia	hy-per-ee'-mee-uh
hyperglycemia	hy-per-gly-see'-me-uh

hypothyroidism	hy-po-thy′-royd-izm
infarction	in-fark′-shun
leukemia	lew-kee′-me-uh
leukocyte	lew′-ko-site
leukopenia	lew-ko-pee′-ne-uh
lymphocyte	limf′-oh-site
macrocyte	mak′-ro-site
metrorrhagia	met-ro-ray′-jee-uh
monocyte	mon′-oh-site
mononucleosis	mon-oh-new-klee-oh′-sis
myocarditis	my-oh-kar-die′-tis
neutropenia	new-tro-pee′-ne-uh
occlusion	ok-klew′-shun
parenteral	pair-en′-ter-al
paroxysmal tachycardia	pair-ox-iz′-mal tak-kee-kar′-de-uh
patent ductus arteriosus	pay′-tent duk′-tus ar-tear-ee-oh′-sus
pericarditis	pear-eh-kar-die′-tis
pericardiectomy	pear-eh-kar-de-ek′-to-me
pericardium	pear-eh-kar′-de-um
periosteum	pear-ee-oss′-te-um
phlebitis	flee-bye′-tis
rhinorrhagia	rine-oh-ray′-jee-uh
sphygmomanometer	sfig-mo-man-om′-me-ter
stenosis	sten-oh′-sis
systolic	sis-toll′-ik
tachyphasia	tak-kee-faz′-ee-uh
tachypnea	tak-ip′-nee-uh
thrombosis	throm-bo′-sis
thrombus	throm′-bus
urostasis	you-ro-stay′-sis
valvotomy	val-vot′-oh-me
vena cava	vee′-na kay′-va
ventricle	ven′-trik-ull
venule	ven′-yule

REVIEW TEST:
THE CARDIOVASCULAR AND CIRCULATORY SYSTEMS

1.   What vessels carry blood away from the heart?

2.   What vessels carry blood to the heart?

3.   Name five components of blood.

4.   Name the four chambers of the heart.

5.   Differentiate between arteriosclerosis and atherosclerosis.

6.   Differentiate between diastolic and systolic.

7.   Differentiate between bradycardia and tachycardia.

8.   Define hypertension.

9.   Define hemostasis.

10.   Define myocarditis.

11.   Define aneurysm.

12.   Define aorta.

13.   Give term for enlarged heart.

14.   Give term for white blood cells.

15.   Give term for blood in urine.

16.   Give term for abnormally rapid breathing.

17.   Give term for hemorrhage from the nose.

18.   Differentiate between endocarditis and pericarditis.

19.   Define hyperglycemia.

20.   Define erythrocytosis.

5

THE NERVOUS SYSTEM

While other systems are complicated, the nervous system is the most complicated in the human body. The nervous system is the body's adaptive and adjusting machinery; it may be thought of as a computer, since stimuli are received and messages carried to and from the brain, controlling all parts of the body. There are actually three systems, and we will deal with each one separately. We will also study the eye and ear along with the nervous system since they are so closely related.

Central Nervous System (CNS)

This consists of the brain and the nerves of the spinal column. The brain receives and sends out messages to every cell in the body through various types of *neurons* (see Fig. 5). In a nerve cell, the *axon* is the carrying-toward part and the *dendrite* is the carrying-away part. The fibers of these cells are coated with a sheath of fatty tissue called *myelin,* which acts as insulation.

The brain, enclosed within the hard shell of the skull, has an area called the *medulla* which controls rhythmic motions of the body, including breathing. Another area, the *cerebellum,* controls coordination of muscular activity. Another area, the *cerebrum,* controls all man's *conscious* acts.

The exposed human brain resembles a maze of lumps, coils, and bumps, yet this three pounds of living tissue is the storage unit for memory and learning, motivator of all behavior, and controller of blood cells, body temperature, blood sugar, breathing, sight, sound and smell, taste and touch, and hormone production. In addition, it sorts and processes information, impressions, and sensory signals. The brain makes up only 2% of body weight but uses 1/6 of the output of the heart and 1/5 of the body's oxygen. It contains 10 billion nerve cells which manage a communications system to and from every cell in the body, through 86 major nerves and hundreds of thousands of smaller nerves. The brain operates on 20 watts of electrical energy, generated by nerve cells that act like tiny dynamos, producing electricity from the chemical fuel of the body's supply of glucose and oxygen.

The brain is a "double" organ, the control center in each half controlling the opposite half of the body. Normally, connections between the two halves permit an exchange of information. However, if the connections between the two halves must be severed surgically, each half can perform as a separate brain, each with its own memory and will. Memories stored in one half are not available to the other half, but the "split" brain can be trained to handle such a situation.

Research on the brain is progressing in two areas: scientists are studying brain damage, disorders of the nervous system, and mental illnesses, while educators are concerned with learning processes and memory. Electrical stimulation is now used to study causes of mental illness, and mood-changing drugs are used for emotional disorders. Electrosurgery, used to destroy certain nerve cells, is helping greatly in the treatment of such diseases as epilepsy, schizophrenia, and Parkinson's disease. Brain surgery is being refined by "geographical mapping" of all the regions in the brain. The discovery of DNA and RNA is helping to crack the genetic code of the brain; present evidence suggests that 40% of all neurological disorders may be hereditary or chemical in orgin. Under the influence of certain chemicals, male animals build nests and act as if they were mothers; brave animals become cowards; timid animals become brave. Apparently, our drives and emotions can be completely reversed by changes in brain chemistry.

In another 15 years, scientists may know how the brain works to cause us to think. They may be able to correct neuroses and psychoses; and they probably will know what factors control personality. Thus we are finding the missing links to emotional reactions, the basis of our awareness of the world, and an account for almost every facet of human behavior.

THE PARTS OF THE BRAIN

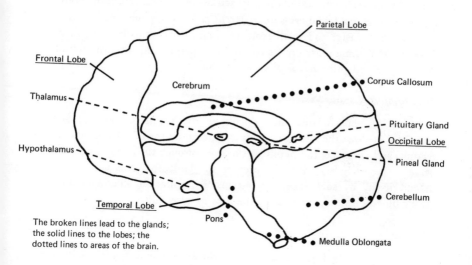

Frontal Lobe

Parietal Lobe

Cerebrum

Corpus Callosum

Thalamus

Pituitary Gland

Occipital Lobe

Hypothalamus

Pineal Gland

Cerebellum

Temporal Lobe

Pons

The broken lines lead to the glands;
the solid lines to the lobes; the
dotted lines to areas of the brain.

Medulla Oblongata

THE PARTS OF A NERVE CELL (NEURON)

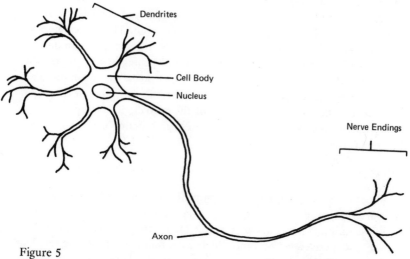

Dendrites

Cell Body

Nucleus

Nerve Endings

Axon

Figure 5

Pheripheral Nervous System

This system is composed of 12 pairs of *cranial nerves* and 31 pairs of *spinal nerves*. *Afferent* nerves carry sensations to the brain *from* the body, e.g., pain, heat, cold, and pressure. *Efferent* nerves carry such sensations as sight, hearing, taste, and smell from the brain to the muscles. The short distance from these sense organs to the brain permits rapid transmittal of messages; this adaption has great survival value.

Autonomous Nervous System

This system controls such organs as the stomach, kidneys, and intestines. It slows the heart or speeds it up, empties the bladder, clears the rectum, and contracts the pupils of the eyes through the *parasympathetic nerves*. The *sympathetic nerves* prepare the body for crisis in order to defend itself, by such means as increasing respiration, dilating pupils, raising blood pressure, and starting the flow of adrenalin.

The Eye

Looking at Fig. 6A, you can see that the eye is connected to the brain by the *optic nerve,* which furnishes the *retina* of the eye with a layer of cells that react to light. The optic nerve and eyeball can be pictured as a cord attached to the back of the brain, extending to the face, with a bulb on the end of the cord. The *rods* and *cones* are nerve cells lining the inner retina. The *rods* in the retina react to white light, and the *cones* react to colored light. The *lens* is the focusing mechanism. The *iris* enlarges or contracts according to the degree of brightness, regulating the amount of light which strikes the retina. The *pupil* is the opening which admits light. *Aqueous* and *vitreus humors* are liquids which keep the eye moistened. The *choroid coat* keeps out all light but that entering through the pupil. The *sclera* is the tough white coating of the eyeball, protecting the eye to some degree. The *cornea* is an inner five-layer coating under the sclera, covering the eye.

The Ear

Looking at Fig. 6B, note the following parts of the ear: The *pinna* is the curved bowl of the outer ear which collects sound waves to be carried to the eardrum. The *eardrum* is a membrane stretched across the ear to receive sound waves and transmit them to the bones of the middle ear. The *malleus* (hammer) is in direct contact with the eardrum; the *incus* (anvil)

THE EYE

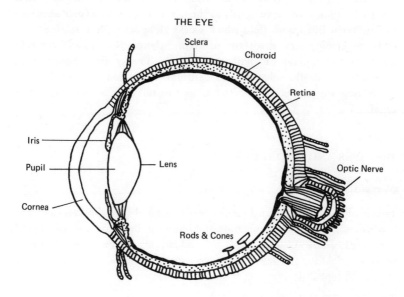

THE EAR

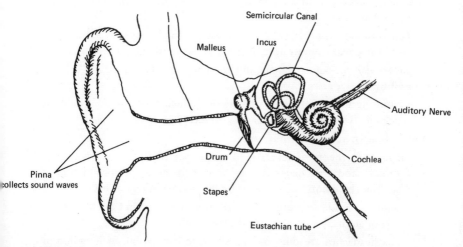

Figure 6

makes contact with the stapes; the *stapes* (stirrup) touches the membrane over the opening to the inner ear. Within the inner ear, the *auditory nerve* turns vibrations into nerve signals to the brain. The *cochlea* (snail shell) is a hollow canal filled with fluid which works along with the *eustachian tube* and the *semicircular canal* to maintain balance. The eustachian tube connects the middle ear with the throat, allowing air pressure to be equalized on both sides of the eardrum. Sensations of dizziness or seasickness can sometimes be traced to a disturbance in the semicircular canal.

DISEASES AND DISORDERS

Nervous System

Encephalitis. This is a broad name covering a number of diseases caused by a virus which creates inflammation and lesions in the brain and spinal cord; the diseases are characterized by sudden high fever, convulsions or muscular rigidity, and involuntary movements. "Sleeping sickness" is one type of encephalitis.

Epilepsy. There are four types:

Grand mal produces severe convulsions and unconsciousness after the seizure has passed. Patients usually sense when a seizure is about to occur, become restless, and as the seizure begins the person loses control and falls, going into convulsions.

Petit mal is a simple lapse of consciousness which lasts only a minute or two. The person almost never realizes he has been unconscious at all.

Jacksonian produces tremors, but the patient walks, talks, and behaves as if under hypnosis.

Febrile occurs in infants as the result of high fever. If the child has repeated attacks, grand mal may be suspected.

Headaches. There are also four types:

Migraine is the most severe kind, accompanied by nausea, vomiting, dizziness, and great pain. It may be caused by an overproduction of histamine, by emotional stress, or by dilation of a brain artery.

Histamine headaches usually occur over one eye and are the direct result of an overproduction of histamine.

Sinus headaches are due to congestion, inflammation, or infection of one or more sinus cavities in the head. Infection in the frontal sinuses causes the most severe pain.

Psychogenic are nervous or tension headaches, the result of worry, stress, overwork, lack of oxygen, smoking or drinking too much, or even too much coffee. These are the most common headaches.

Herpes zoster. Commonly called "shingles." This is an acute infection of the central nervous system, caused by a virus, and characterized by neuralgic pain with a skin rash that is difficult to cure. *Herpes Simplex* is a skin rash marked by clusters of watery blisters. *Herpes* denotes a number of skin rashes.

Hiccups. Involuntary spasmodic contraction of the diaphragm.

Meningitis. A broad term indicating inflammation of a membrane. The best known type is *spinal* meningitis, marked by a high fever, pain in the back and legs, and sometimes paralysis.

Neuritis. Inflammation of one or more nerves with pain and tenderness at the affected area. This is usually a temporary ailment, relieved by aspirin and heat, although there are 56 different kinds of neuritis, some more serious than others.

Parkinson's disease. A progressive disease marked by a masklike face, tremors and weakness of muscles, and shaking palsy.

Sciatica. Severe pain in the leg along the route of the sciatic nerve, affecting the muscles of the calf of the leg — may be caused by a back injury, hip damage, diabetes, or a vitamin deficiency.

Strokes. There are four types:

Embolus is caused by a clot breaking away from its point of origin and cutting off circulation at some place in the brain. This type is usually accompanied by sudden, acutely severe headache. There may be partial or complete paralysis or none at all.

Hemorrhage is cerebrovascular accident, with hemorrhage at some place in the brain; it may occur when a person is awake, and involves only one side of the body as a rule.

Subarachnoid is the athlete's stroke, caused by an accident while engaged in some exertion. It is very severe and usually fatal, due to massive hemorrhage in the brain.

Thrombus is caused by a blood clot somewhere in the brain; this type can occur when a person is asleep and wakes to find his body paralyzed.

Tics. Involuntary spasms of a nerve; can occur anywhere in the body, but is common in the face, around the eye or mouth.

Trigeminal neuralgia (also called tic doloreaux). Severe attacks of pain in the area of the trigeminal nerve, around the eye, upper and lower jaw, and temple.

The Eye

Astigmatism. A defective curvature of the refractive surface of the eye, causing focus to be inaccurate — corrected with glasses.

Blindness. There are about 25 types of blindness, and several degrees of blindness. Some so-called "blind" people can see outlines of shapes when in bright light, some have peripheral vision (to the sides) but not direct vision straight ahead. Some blind people can see well enough to get around but not well enough to read. Blindness may be present at birth or caused by some damage later. Also, temporary or even permanent blindness may be caused by hysteria — some psychic shock, such as witnessing a murder, which causes the person unconsciously not to want to see.

Cataracts. There are more than 50 different kinds of cataracts, but in general, the term means a clouding over of the lens of the eye, obstructing passage of light. This is sometimes due to shock or injury, sometimes due to old age, or may develop in connection with some other disease.

Conjunctivitis. Inflammation of the conjunctiva (the delicate membrane that lines the eyelids and covers the eyeball); may be caused by overexposure to ultraviolet light, hay fever or other allergy, or bacteria.

Detached retina. A serious condition in which the retina becomes detached from its anchorage to the iris and can be the cause of blindness if not immediately and properly treated. The patient with a detached retina may be rehabilitated by placing his head between sandbags and covering the eyes, thus lying completely still and not using the eye for several weeks while the eye heals. Also, there are surgical methods of repair, such as photocoagulation with lasers. The condition may not be curable if caused by an accident and subsequent damage to the retina.

hardening of the eye, resulting in blindness if not properly cared for. Medications in the form of eye drops containing adrenalin and histamine, dropped into the eye faithfully at specified periods, can slow down the deterioration process of glaucoma.

Hyperopia. Commonly called far-sightedness, due to a lack of sufficient refracting power in focusing; corrected with glasses.

Myopia. Commonly called near-sightedness, due to too great refractive power in focusing; corrected with glasses.

Strabismus. Called cock-eyed, this is due to a deviation of the eyes so that one eye may look straight ahead, the other off to one side. Cross-eyed people are suffering from a severe kind of strabismus. Most patients with strabismus can have the condition corrected by glasses or surgery.

The Ear

Deafness. There are about 30 kinds of deafness, attributable to infection, organic diseases, damage, calcification, and psychic or hysterical reaction. There are also degrees of deafness, from the inability to distinguish tones to total deafness. Some types of deafness can be cured: psychic, by psychiatric treatment; calcification, by surgery; infections, by antibiotics.

Ear infections. These are many and varied also; they can be caused by bacteria, by injury, or by such things as trying to clean out ear wax using a pencil, a wire, or other material which may be covered with bacteria. Most can be treated with antibiotics.

Labyrinthitis. (also called otitis interna). Inflammation of the labyrinth or internal portion of the ear. This sometimes causes dizziness, and imbalance like that experienced with trouble in the semicircular canal.

Otitis media. Inflammation of the middle ear, the area between the eardrum and the semicircular canal.

Tympanotomy. Commonly called "punctured eardrum." This is often the result of an infection in the middle ear which has caused the doctor to lance the eardrum to permit pus to drain. People may puncture their own eardrums by improper probing to clean out ear wax.

TERMINOLOGY

Roots	Terms	Descriptions
aud —, aur— *oto—* ear, hearing	audio/meter ot/itis media	instrument to measure hearing inflammation of the middle ear
blepharo— eyelid	blephar/itis blepharo/rrhaphy	inflammation of the eyelid suturing the eyelid
cerebro— brain	cerebro/ocular cerebr/otomy	pertaining to brain and eyes surgical incision into brain
cort— covering, bark	cort/ico/tropic cerebral cortex	affecting the adrenal cortex outer covering of the brain
dacry— tear duct	dacry/aden/itis dacryo/rrhea	inflammation of a tear duct constantly watering eyes

Roots	Terms	Descriptions
iri—	irido/plegia	paralysis of the eye's iris
iris	irido/cele	hernia of the iris of the eye
kerat—	kerat/oma	tumor of the cornea of the eye
cornea	kerato/hemia	deposit of blood in the cornea
neuro—	neur/asthenia	nervous exhaustion, weakness
nerve	neuro/fibr/oma	fibrous tumor of nerve tissue
ocul—	oculo/spinal	pertaining to the eye and spine
ophthal—	ophthalm/ologist	specialist in eye diseases
eye		
phren—	phreno/plegia	paralysis of mental faculties
mind	phren/asthenia	weak-mindedness; idiocy
psych—	psycho/genic	originating in the mind
mind	psych/otic	a severe mental disorder

Additional Vocabulary

autonomic: that part of the nervous system which is functionally independent, self-controlling

Babinski-Weil: a test for balance (also called Barany's finger-nose test). The patient stands on one foot, arms extended, eyes closed, then tries to touch the end of his nose with the tip of his index finger.

cerebellum: that part of the brain which controls coordination of body movements

cerebrum: the main part of the brain occupying the upper part of the cranium, forming the largest part of the central nervous system

choroid: the covering of the eye which nourishes the retina and the lens

CNS: abbreviation for central nervous system

CVA: abbreviation for cerebrovascular accident, a stroke

ECT/EST: electroshock therapy, used to treat mental patients

EEG: electroencephalogram, an electrical-impulse picture of the brain waves

euphoria: a feeling of well-being and bodily comfort

febrile: with fever, an elevated temperature

grand mal: literally, great sickness — a form of epilepsy (see petit mal)

hypothalamus: the part of the brain which controls visceral activities, water balance, sleep, and to a degree, temperature (when there is no fever from disease)

lacrimal: pertaining to the tear ducts and tears

lesion: any break of tissue or loss of function of any body part; not necessarily a wound

malaise: a feeling of illness, depression, or body discomfort

olfactory: pertaining to the nerve (olfactory) which activates the sense of smell

petit mal: little sickness — another milder form of epilepsy

pineal: the pineal gland in the brain, so named because it is shaped like a pine cone

pons: the part of the brain lying nearest the six pair of nerves which act as a transmitter of sensations from the cerebellum

temporal: the lobe of the brain which lies nearest the temples

vertigo: a feeling of dizziness, as when the room seems to whirl

Pronunciations and Accents for Terms

afferent	af´-fer-ent
anastomosis	an-as-to-mo´-sis
aqueous	ak´-wee-us
astigmatism	ah-stig´-ma-tizm
audiometer	aw-dee-ah´-meter
autonomic	au-ton´-oh-mik
axon	aks´-on
Babinski—Weil	Bab-in´-skee Wile
blepharitis	blef-ar-eye´-tis
blepharorrhaphy	blef-ar-orr´-oh-fee
cerebellum	ser-eh-bell´-um
cerebral cortex	seer-ee´-bral kor´-tex
cerebro-ocular	seer-ee´-bro-ok´-you-lar
cerebrotomy	seer-ee-brot´-oh-me
cerebrum	seer-ee´-brum
choroid	kore´-oyd
cochlea	koke´-lee-uh
conjunctiva	kon-junk´-ti-vah

(continued)

Pronunciations and Accents for Terms (continued)

conjunctivitis	kon-junk-ti-vye'-tis
cornea	kor'-nee-uh
corpus callosum	kor'-pus kal-oh'-sum
corticotropic	kor-ti-trow'-pik
dacryadenitis	dak-ree-add-en-eye'-tis
dacryorrhea	dak-ree-oh-ree'-uh
dendrite	den'-drite
embolus	em'-bo-lus
encephalitis	en-sef-uh-lie'-tis
endotoxin	en-do-tok'-sin
euphoria	you-for'-ee-uh
eustachian	you-stak'-ee-en
febrile	fee'-brile
fibroma	fy-bro'-mah
glaucoma	glaw-ko'-mah
grand mal	grand mahl
herpes zoster	her'-peez zos'-ter
histamine	his'-tah-meen
hypothalamus	hy-po-thal'-ah-mus
incus	ink'-us
iridoplegia	ear-rid-oh-play'-jee-uh
ischemia	is-kee'-me-ah
keratocele	ker-rat'-oh-seal
keratohemia	ker-rat-oh-hee'-me-uh
keratoma	ker-ah-to'-mah
lacrimal	lak'-reh-mal
malaise	mal-ayz'
malleus	mal'-ee-us
medulla	meh-dull'-ah
myelin	my'-eh-lin
neurasthenia	new-ras-thee'-ne-uh
neurofibroma	new-ro-fi-brow'-mah
neuron	new'-ron
oculospinal	ok-you-lo-spy'-nal
olfactory	all-fak'-to-ree
ophthalmologist	off-thal-mol'-oh-gist
otitis media	oh-ty'-tis mee'-de-ah
parasympathetic	pair-ah-sim-pa-thet'-ik

parietal	pair-eye´-ah-tal
peripheral	per-if´-er-al
petit mal	pe´-teh mahl
phrenasthenia	fren-as-thee´-ne-uh
phrenoplegia	fren-oh-play´-jee-uh
pineal	pin´-ee-al
pinna	pin´-nah
pons	ponz
psychogenic	sigh-ko-jen´-ik
psychosomatic	sigh-ko-so-mat´-ik
psychotic	sigh-kot´-ik
retina	ret´-eh-nah
sciatica	sigh-at´-ik-ah
sclera	skler´-ah
sequelae	see-kwel´-eye
stapes	stay´-peez
strabismus	stra-bis´-mus
subarachnoid	sub-air-ak´-noyd
temporal	tem´-por-al
thalamus	thal´-ah-mus
thrombus	throm´-bus
thymus	thy´-mus
trigeminal	try-jem´-eh-nal
neuralgia	new-ral´-jee-uh
vertigo	ver´-teh-go
vitreous	vit´-ree-us

REVIEW TEST: THE NERVOUS SYSTEM

1. Name four lobes of the brain.

2. Name two glands in the brain.

3. Name three parts of the eye.

4. Name three parts of the ear.

5. Define iritis.

6. Define strabismus.

7. Define dacryadenitis.

8. Define neurofibroma.

9. Define blepharorrhaphy.

10. Name two types of epilepsy.

11. Name two types of strokes.

12. Differentiate between cornea and cochlea.

13. Differentiate between cerebrotomy and craniotomy.

14. Give the term for a herniated iris.

15. Give the term for inflammation of an eyelid.

16. Give the term for tumor of the cornea.

17. Give the term for far-sightedness.

18. Give the term for near-sightedness.

19. What does the cerebellum control?

20. What does the cerebrum control?

6

THE REPRODUCTIVE AND URINARY SYSTEMS

REPRODUCTIVE SYSTEM

Female Reproductive System

The internal organs of the female reproductive system are the *ovaries,* two small oval bodies about 1½ inches long and 1 inch wide. The *ova,* or eggs, are produced in the ovaries and stored there. One or more ova are released approximately every 28 days, from one ovary or the other, but not from both at the same period. Each ovary opens into a *fallopian tube* down which the egg proceeds to the *uterus,* a pear-shaped organ about 3 inches long and 2 inches wide when normal size. The open end of the neck of the uterus is the *cervix.* The *vagina* is the area from the cervix to the body opening and is the birth canal. Both the uterus and the cervix, as well as the vagina, are highly elastic and can stretch to more than seven times their normal size when birth is imminent. The uterus, of course, expands continually during pregnancy as the baby grows.

Ovulation, release of an ovum from the ovary, occurs just prior to the menstrual period. The ovum (normally) travels down the fallopian tube into the uterus, where it remains for about five days. If the ovum is fertilized by a sperm cell during this period, pregnancy results. If no fertilization takes place, the ovum dies and is washed out of the uterus as part of the menstrual flow.

If pregnancy occurs, the sperm cell and ovum are united in the uterus within a thin membranous bag called the *amniotic sac.* The sac fills with amniotic fluid in which the fertilized ovum, or *embryo*, lives and grows. The embryo, as it begins to grow, is accompanied by the *placenta*, a cakelike mass which maintains sustenance for the embryo through the *umbilical cord*, a tube which carries the blood supply from the mother.

A baby is termed an embryo to the eighth week of pregnancy, and then a *fetus* from this period until birth. A pregnancy which is not completed is called an *abortion* up to the 16th week, an *immature delivery* up to the 28th week, and a *premature birth* from the 28th to the 36th week. The weight of an embryo at 8 weeks is 4-5 ounces; at the 6th month, about 1 pound; almost all of the weight is added in the 8th and 9th months.

When the fetus has reached full term at the end of nine months or 266 days, the amniotic sac must rupture or be broken by the obstetrician's scalpel, to empty the amniotic fluid to make room for the baby. After the baby is born, the placenta — commonly called the afterbirth — is expelled.

Male Reproductive System

The internal male reproductive system consists of the *prostate gland, seminal vesicles, vas deferens, spermatic cord, epididymis,* and *ejaculatory ducts.* The external system consists of the *testes* (testicles), covered by the *scrotum,* and the *penis.* The prostate is an accessory gland which lies just below the bladder. The seminal vesicles and ejaculatory ducts empty into the prostate. The seminal vesicles, each about the size and shape of the little finger, are located behind the bladder. These secrete the alkaline portion of the seminal fluid. The ejaculatory ducts are formed above the base of the prostate and partially regulate the ejaculation of seminal fluid (semin) through the penis. The testes are egg-shaped glands lying one on either side, behind and slightly below the penis; these glands produce innumerable sperm cells.

DISEASES AND MALFORMATIONS

Female

Amenorrhea. Absence of menstruation, or scanty menstrual flow.

Cysts. Ovarian cysts are quite common in women, often numerous, and may be small or large. They can also occur in the uterus. They cause little trouble unless they begin to grow, and must then be removed because of the likelihood of their causing cancer.

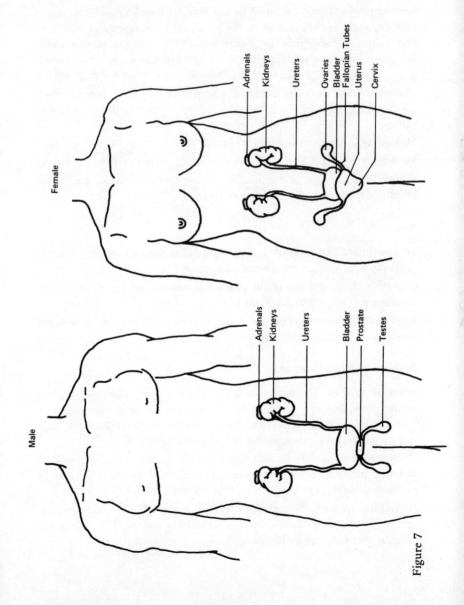

Figure 7

Dysmenorrhea. Painful menstruation, accompanied by cramps.

Ectopic pregnancy. Any pregnancy occurring outside the uterus, usually in one of the fallopian tubes; rarely they have been known to occur in the ovaries or even in the abdomen. Ectopic means "out of place."

Endometriosis. Tissue identical to the mucous membrane of the uterus may grow outside the uterus in the pelvic cavity; it resembles adhesions and causes chronic pain or discomfort. After menopause this tissue atrophies and ceases to cause trouble. It can bleed at a menstrual period, just as the endometrium in the uterus bleeds.

Fibroid tumors. Both the ovaries and uterus are subject to tumors which are thick, ropy masses. Such tumors are suspect because they can lead to cancer.

Menorrhagia. Abnormally heavy menstrual flow.

Metrorrhagia. Hemorrhage from the uterus; not related to menstruation.

Mittelschmerz. "Pain in the middle" − not in the stomach, but in the middle of the month when ovulation occurs.

Male

Cryptorchidism. Undescended testes; they fail to descend into the scrotum − usually occurs about the time of puberty.

Prostatitis. Inflammation of the prostate, often causing interference with urination and inflammation of the bladder.

Syphilis and gonorrhea. Venereal diseases, common to both sexes; both are now curable by antibiotics.

Developmental Abnormalities

Hermaphroditism. The hermaphrodite usually strongly resembles one sex or the other, but may actually be opposite the sex he or she resembles. The true hermaphrodite possesses both male and female sex organs. Now surgery and hormone therapy can correct the condition.

Homosexuality. Modern science still is not certain whether this condition is due to physical causes or emotional imbalance. Early home life may be partly responsible. The word means "love of the same sex."

Impotence. In both the male and female, impotence or frigidity may be due to psychological causes, or to a lack of sex hormones. If due to the latter, it may be cured by hormone therapy.

Sterility. In females, sterility is due to an inability to produce ova, or a stoppage of the fallopian tubes so that ova cannot reach the uterus. In males, the condition is due to an inability to produce sperm cells. Sterility can sometimes be cured by hormone therapy.

In both the male and female, certain sexual functions diminish as a natural result of aging. In women, the time at which menstruation ceases — usually between age 46 and 50 — is called menopause. The diminishing of sexual activity in the male is called *climacteric,* and occurs at about the same age as menopause.

NOTE: Terminology, additional vocabulary, pronunciations and accents applicable to the reproductive system follow The Urinary System.

THE URINARY SYSTEM

The urinary system is made up of organs concerned with production and excretion of urine, which carries wastes from the body, and consists of the *kidneys, ureters, bladder,* and *urethra.* The functions of the urinary system are to eliminate toxic substances, maintain proper water balance in the body, maintain the proper concentration of salts and alkalines in the blood, and keep a proper balance of acids in body fluids.

The kidneys are a pair of organs, lying one on each side of the vertebral column above the two upper lumbar vertebrae. They are usually embedded in a mass of fatty tissue, for protection. Each kidney is about 5 inches long, 3 inches wide, and is soft and pliable.

Blood enters the kidneys through the *renal arteries* and is processed to remove the substances that make up urine. The kidneys are a mass of arteries, veins, capillaries, and lymphatic vessels. Blood is filtered through capillary walls; blood pressure provides the force for this filtration. One-fourth of the total blood supply is filtered through each kidney each minute. The average amount of urine excreted in a 24-hour period is between 3 and 4 pints. A high-protein diet will decrease urine volume; large amounts of water intake increase the volume; strenuous activity also results in less urine output because the body uses some of the fluid for perspiration.

Urine is made up of ammonia, calcium, magnesium, sulphuric acid, phosphoric acid, potassium chloride, sodium chloride, fatty acids, urea, hormones, and water. Ammonia and the minerals potassium chloride, sodium chloride and salts of calcium and magnesium as well as phosphorous and fats in the form of acids are found in the urine along with urea and water. The amount of urea which may be found in blood is referred to as blood urea nitrogen, or BUN. BUN tests are an important diagnostic aid.

Urine is light amber in color and is usually clear. Urine should have a pH, or degree of acidity, of about 6.0.

When urine is excreted from the kidneys, it flows down the ureters to the bladder, where it is stored. While urine is accumulating, the bladder muscles are relaxed to adjust to the volume of fluid. When about one cup of fluid has collected in the bladder, it begins to contract, sphincter muscles open, and urine flows through the urethra to be discharged.

Since water balance is of vital importance to the body, and since the kidneys play a major role in water balance, it is interesting to note the ways by which water is lost, and the amounts. Water is lost through the skin in the amount of about 1 cup; through the lungs, about ½ cup; through the kidneys, between 6 and 8 cups; and through the feces, about ¼ cup. Excessive sweating, vomiting, diarrhea, and blood loss all contribute to loss of water in the body.

The Artificial Kidney Machine

About 100,000 people die each year from kidney diseases. It is estimated that three million Americans have undiagnosed kidney diseases. The artificial kidney machine can and has saved many lives, by replacing the action of kidneys which are failing. This is how it works: A vein and an artery, usually both in one arm, are surgically exposed by a cut-down, and a cannula (tube) inserted which is then connected to the machine. The artificial kidney machine is attached to the artery, the patient's blood flows through the machine, and after completing the machine circuit it flows back into the body by way of the vein. There is a cellophane coil in the machine that contains many "pores" so tiny that only a single molecule of salt and water can pass through. The blood circulates through this coil to be purified and to reduce the concentration of urea. The procedure takes 4-6 hours and is usually repeated 3-4 times weekly. The artificial kidney machine is also used for patients awaiting kidney transplants, maintaining good body function until a transplant is available. The process which the artificial kidney machine performs is called *dialysis*. Patients may go to a hospital for dialysis, but machines are now made that can be used in the home with proper instructions, making treatment available on a larger scale.

Kidney Dialysis Vocabulary

arrhythmia: disturbance of heart rhythm — may be caused by or can be a symptom of kidney disease

A-V shunt: arterial-venous shunt, which consists of a short piece of plastic tubing surgically inserted to connect an artery to a vein, usually placed in the arm so the patient can move about.

casts: cells, fats, and proteins which solidify to the shape of the kidney's tubules and are flushed out with the urine.

dialysate: the saline (salt) solution used in the kidney machine

dialysis:

hemodialysis is the process of circulating blood on one side of a semipermeable membrane while the other side is bathed in the dialysate solution. The toxic products dialyze out of the blood into the dialysis solution.

peritoneal dialysis is the process of allowing external fluid to flow in and out of the peritoneal cavity (abdomen) by way of a dialysis catheter.

dialyzer: the machine itself. There are two types: the coil or Kolff, and the parallel-flow or Kiil. The coil type is preferred in most dialysis centers.

diuretic: a medication which takes fluid out of body tissues and thus increases the output of urine

edema: excess fluid in body tissues, causing swelling

electrolytes: the salts in the blood, generally referred to as Na (sodium), K (potassium), Cl (chloride), and CO_2 (carbon dioxide)

fistula: arterio-venous lump formed surgically by connecting an artery to a vein under the skin. This type of fistula is the result of the subcutaneous connection of the artery and vein. True fistulas are abnormal passages from inside the body to the surface.

glomeruli: capillary clusters of tiny blood vessels in the kidney which filter the blood to form urine

glomerulonephritis, acute: inflammation involving the glomeruli, causing marked decrease in the rate at which fluid which makes up urine is separated or filtered from blood

glomerulonephritis, chronic: a slow, progressive damage to the glomeruli, resulting in uremia

hemolysis: breakdown of red blood cells, occurring in some types of kidney disease

isotonic: a solution containing the same concentration of salts as plasma; equality of osmotic pressure between two different solutions

nephrolithiasis: presence of calculi (stones) in the kidneys, causing decreased kidney function

nephron: a filtering unit and associated tubule found throughout the kidneys

nephrosclerosis: hardening of the arteries of the kidneys, causing decreased kidney function

nephrosis: a disease within the kidneys apparent by loss of protein in large amounts

polycystic kidney disease: a condition in which many small cysts are found within the kidneys, causing malfunction

pyelonephritis: inflammation of the pelvic bowl of the kidney due to bacterial infection

renal failure, acute: the kidneys fail to function after injury or ingestion of poison. If the patient can be kept alive, the kidneys may repair themselves while the artificial kidney machine takes over for them.

renal failure, chronic: permanent loss of kidney function. The artificial kidney machine is then used regularly to maintain life

renal tubular acidosis: excessive acid content in the blood because it cannot be removed by the failing kidneys

urea: a nitrogen end-product of protein metabolism

uremic poisoning: a severe illness due to urine in the blood, with accompanying nausea, vomiting, twitching, lethargy, and death

uropathies: any disease of the urinary tract which affects the kidneys

DISEASES

Acetonuria. Acetone, an acid solvent, shows up in the urine when excessive amounts of fats have been eaten or when fats have not been properly broken down by the kidneys. Acetone is produced during starvation, when the body burns its own stored fat.

Albuminuria. The presence of abnormal amounts of albumin in the urine, regarded as evidence of kidney disease; particularly dangerous during pregnancy.

Cystitis. Inflammation of the bladder.

Dysuria. Painful or difficult urination, a symptom of some disease or disorder in the urinary system.

Enuresis. Bed-wetting; may be due to faulty toilet training, to some psychological or emotional disturbance, or rarely to some physical disorder.

Glycosuria. Apart from being a symptom of diabetes, abnormal amounts of sugar in the urine can be caused by an excessive intake of sweets, or by what is known as emotional glycosuria, due to overactivity of the adrenal glands.

Hematuria. Blood in the urine; may be caused by infection in the kidneys or elsewhere in the urinary tract, by injury to the kidney or bladder, or by a growth in the urinary system.

Incontinence. The inability to retain urine; may be due to lack of sphincter-muscle tone; most often seen in old, ill patients.

Kidney stones. Properly called *renal calculi*. Small stones are usually passed, but larger ones may lodge somewhere in the kidney, ureter, or bladder and cause renal colic with intense, spasmodic pain.

Nephritis. Inflammation of one or both kidneys; may be acute or chronic

Pyelitis. Inflammation of the pelvic bowl of the kidney.

Urethritis. Inflammation of the urethra, caused by highly acid urine, the presence of bacteria, or constriction of the urethral passage.

TERMINOLOGY APPLICABLE TO THE REPRODUCTIVE AND URINARY SYSTEMS

Roots	Terms	Descriptions
cervic— *trachel—* neck	cervic/itis trachelo/rrhaphy	inflammation of the cervix suture of the cervix
colp— vagina	colp/ectasis colpo/plasty	dilation of the vagina plastic surgery on vagina
cyesis— *gravid—* pregnancy	ovario/cyesis primi/gravida	ovarian pregnancy first pregnancy
cyst— *vesic—* bladder, sac	cysto/scopy vesiculo/gram	inspection of the bladder fluoroscope of a vesicle

(continued)

Roots	Terms	Descriptions
gyne— woman	gyneco/genic gyneco/mastia	producing female traits female breasts in a male
hyster— *metro—* uterus	hystero/pexy metro/rrhexis	surgical fixation, uterus rupture of the uterus
mamm— *mast—* breast	mamm/ectomy mast/algia	surgical removal of breast pain in the breast
lacto— milk	lacta/tion lacto/toxin	secretion of milk in breasts toxic substance in milk
meno— menses	a/meno/rrhea meno/rrhagia	scant or no menstruation excessive menstrual flow
natus— birth	pre/natal post/natal	occurring before birth occurring after birth
nephro— *ren—*	nephro/litho/tripsy renal colic	crushing of kidney stones severe pain in the kidney
oophor— *ovario—* ovary	oophoro/cyst/ectomy ovario/cele	removal of ovarian cyst hernia of an ovary
orchi— testes	orchio/pexy orchio/plasty	fixing testes in scrotum plastic surgery on testes
ovi— (egg)	ovi/duct	tube which egg passes through
part— labor, production	ovi/parity part/uri/tion	production of ova giving birth
pyelo— kidney pelvis	pyelo/lith/ectomy pyel/ectasis	removal of kidney stone dilation of kidney pelvis
semin— (seed)	in/semin/ation	introduction of semen
thel— (nipple)	thel/itis	inflammation of a nipple
uria— urine	glycos/uria hemat/uria	sugar in the urine blood in the urine

Additional Vocabulary

calculi: calcifications or stones — can be present in the bladder, kidney, salivary glands, gallbladder, breast, liver, and pancreas

castration: removal of ovaries or testes, making the person sterile — sometimes necessary because of cancer

catheter: tube for giving or withdrawing fluids, as in using a catheter to the bladder to withdraw urine

D & C: dilation and curettage, a procedure used to dilate the uterus to scrape and stop hemorrhage, or to remove an afterbirth which has failed be expelled

episiotomy: surgical slit between the vagina and anus to make childbirth easier

G-U: abbreviation for genito-urinary

leukorrhea: whitish discharge from the vagina, a common gynecological disorder due to irritation or infection

monilia: a fungus, persistent when present in the vagina, anus, or cervix — infectious, often passed back and forth between man and wife

neoplasm: literally, new formation — any new abnormal growth

"Pap" smear: test devised by George Papanicolaou, a Greek doctor. Cancer cells can be detected by swabbing the vagina and placing the smear on a slide under a microscope

speculum: instrument used to widen passages for visual inspection, as in a pelvic examination

teratology: the study of malformations of the fetus, such as those which occurred from the use of thalidomide

uterine cautery: "burning" the neck of the uterus or surface of the uterus with an electric current to kill tissue*

viable: alive, capable of living, as in delivery of a viable infant

---

* Sometimes, after several pregnancies, and often due to tears in the uterus because it failed to enlarge rapidly for birth, the uterus will have scars, nodes, or small growths which are not normal. Uterine cautery is used to eliminate these, and to help prevent future possibility of cancer.

Pronunciations and Accents for Terms

acetonuria	ass-eh-tone-you'-re-uh
albuminuria	al-bu-min-you'-re-uh
amenorrhea	aye-men-oh-ree'-uh
amniotic sac	am-nee-ot-ik sac'
androgen	an'-dro-jen
andosterone	an-doss'-ter-own
anomaly	an-ah'-ma-lee
arrhythmia	air-rith'-me-uh
calculi	kal'-kew-lee
cannula	kan'-you-lah
castration	kas-tray'-shun
catheter	kath'-eh-ter
cervicitis	ser-veh-sigh'-tis
cervix	ser'-vix
colpectasis	kol-peck'-tah-sis
colpoplasty	kol'-po-plas-tee
cryptorchidism	krypt-or'-kid-izm
cyesiology	sigh-ee-zee-ol'-oh-jee
cystitis	sis-ty'-tis
cystoscopy	sis-tos'-ko-pee
dialysate	dy-al'-eh-sate
dialysis	dy-al'-eh-sis
diuretic	dy-you-ret'-ik
dysmenorrhea	dis-men-oh-ree'-uh
dysuria	dis-you'-ree-uh
ectopic	ek-top'-ik
embryo	em'-bree-oh
enuresis	en-you-ree'-sis
endometriosis	en-do-mee-tree-oh'-sis
epididymis	ep-eh-did'-eh-mis
episiotomy	ee-pee-zee-ot'-oh-me
estrogen	ess'-tro-jen
fallopian	fal-low'-pee-un
fetus	fee'-tus
fistula	fiss'-tew-lah
glomerulonephritis	glow-mer-you-lo-ne-fry'-tis
glycosuria	gly-ko-shew'-re-uh
gonorrhea	gon-oh-ree'-uh

gynecogenic	gy-nee-ko-jen´-ik
gynecomastia	gy-nee-ko-mass´-te-uh
hematuria	heem-ah-tew´-re-uh
hermaphroditism	her-maf´-ro-dye-tizm
hysteropexy	hiss-ter´-oh-pex-ee
impotence	im´-po-tense
isotonic	eye-so-ton´-ik
lactation	lak-tay´-shun
lactotoxin	lak´-to-tock-sin
leukorrhea	lew-ko-ree´-uh
mammectomy	mam-mek´-to-me
mastalgia	mass-tal´-jee-uh
menorrhagia	men-oh-raj´-ee-uh
metrorrhagia	met-ro-raj´-ee-uh
metrorrhexis	met-ro-rex´-is
mittelschmerz	mit´-tel-shmerts
monilia	mon-nil´-ee-uh
nephritis	neh-fry´-tis
nephrolithiasis	neh-fro-lith-eye´-uh-sis
nephrolithotripsy	neh-fro-lith´-oh-trip-see
oophorocystectomy	oo-for-oh-sis-tek´-to-me
orchiopexy	or´-kee-oh-peck-see
ovariocele	oh-vair´-ee-oh-seal
ovariocyesis	oh-vair-ee-oh-sigh-ee´-sis
oviduct	oh´-veh-duct
oviparity	oh-veh-pair´-eh-tee
ovulation	oh-vew-lay´-shun
Papanicolaou	Pa-pa-nik´-oh-lau
parturition	par-tur-ih´-shun
peritoneal	pear-eh-to-nee´-ul
placenta	pla-sen´-tah
polycystic	polly-sis´-tik
progesterone	pro-jes´-ter-own
prostate	pros´-tate (*not* prostrate)
prostatitis	pro-stat-eye´-tis
pyelectasis	py-el-ek´-tah-sis
pyelitis	py-el-eye´-tis
pyelolithotomy	py-el-oh-lith-ot´-oh-me
renal	ree´-nal

(continued)

Pronunciations and Accents for Terms (continued)

scrotum	skro'-tum
seminal	sem'-eh-nal
speculum	spek'-you-lum
syphilis	siff'-eh-lis
teratology	tear-ah-tol'-oh-jee
testes	tess'-teez
testosterone	tes-tos'-ter-own
thelitis	thel-eye'-tis
trachelorrhaphy	tray-kel-oh'-raf-ee
umbilical	um-bill'-eh-kal
urea	you-ree'-uh
uremia	you-ree'-me-uh
ureter	you'-reh-ter
urethra	you-ree'-thrah
urethritis	you-ree-thry'-tis
uropathy	you'-ro-pathy
uterus	you'-terus
vagina	vah-jy'-nah
vas deferens	vass deff'-er-enz
venereal	ven-ear'-ee-al
vesiculogram	vess-ik'you-lo-gram
viable	vy'-ah-bal

REVIEW TEST: THE REPRODUCTIVE AND URINARY SYSTEMS

1. Name three diseases of the female reproductive system.

2. Name two diseases of the male reproductive system.

3. Name four diseases of the urinary system.

4. Define adrenalectomy.

5. Define dysmenorrhea.

6. Define nephrosclerosis.

7.   Define endometriosis.

8.   Define cystitis.

9.   Differentiate between menorrhagia and metrorrhagia.

10.   Differentiate between pyelogenic and pyogenic.

11.   Differentiate between hematuria and glycosuria.

12.   Differentiate between hysterectomy and nephrectomy.

13.   What is an ectopic pregnancy?

14.   Give the term for surgical fixation of the uterus.

15.   Give the term for pain in the breast.

16.   Define urostasis.

17.   Define nephromalacia.

18.   Give the term for inspection of the bladder.

19.   Define nephrolithotripsy.

20.   Define metrorrhexis.

7

THE ENDOCRINE SYSTEM

The endocrine system is made up of glands that secrete internally. They are known as ductless glands because they have no ducts or openings. Consult Fig. 8 to locate the following glands:

1. The *pituitary* gland is called the master gland because it regulates thyroid activity, contracts blood vessels, inhibits diuresis (too much secretion of urine), and regulates the other glands of the system. Growth hormones are manufactured here, as well as *thyrotropin,* a hormone controlling some phases of pregnancy and the menstrual cycle, *corticotropin,* (ACTH) which stimulates the adrenal cortex, and *prolactin,* which stimulates the formation of milk in the breasts after childbirth.

2. The *pineal* gland, deep in the brain, is believed to produce histamine and other hormones, but there is still some question as to whether this is really an endocrine gland.

3. The *thyroids* are located in the neck on either side of the trachea, and produce *thyroxin.* If the thyroids are overactive, the person has thin, dry skin and hair, and is usually thin and hyperactive; these are the people who are always "on the go." If the thyroids are underactive, the person has thick, coarse, oily skin and hair, and are often considered lazy. If there is a deficiency of iodine in the diet, goiter results because of an enlargement of the thyroids.

4. The *parathyroids* are located immediately above and below the thyroids, two on each side. They regulate the metabolism of calcium and phosphorus in the body.

5. The *thymus* is located in the thoracic area below the thyroids. At birth this gland is large, but grows smaller and almost disappears by adolescence. Information about the thymus is still scarce; it is believed to have some effect on growth, and recently scientists have discovered that the thymus controls antibodies, produces lymphocytes, and has something to do with the rejection of transplants in the body.

6. The *adrenals* are two small glands which sit upon the kidneys (*ad* = toward or on, *renal* = kidney). These glands weigh only about ¼ ounce each, yet they produce about 50 hormones and substances similar to hormones that are vital to life.

   The adrenals produce *adrenalin,* the hormone which supports the body in times of fear, anger, or crisis. Adrenalin (epinephrine) increases heart rate, speeds the rate of blood circulation and raises blood pressure. This permits a person to be stronger, run faster, and fight harder than would be normal for him. The cortex (covering) of the adrenals produce *steroid hormones* (similar to cortisone) which regulate metabolism of fats, proteins, and carbohydrates. Another substance produced by the adrenals helps to control the body's balance of water and minerals, and another initiates production of some of the sex hormones.

   Without these substances, a human could not live more than a few days: blood pressure would drop alarmingly, appetite would lessen, weight loss would be great, and death would follow. Fortunately, if the adrenals fail to function or must be removed, synthetic hormones can now be provided, thanks to scientific progress. To keep the adrenals healthy, we should attempt to maintain ourselves on an even keel emotionally; anger, fear, and stress are damaging to these glands.

7. The pancreas, lying behind the stomach near the spleen, is the largest of the endocrines. It secretes *insulin* and *glucagon* to break down carbohydrates and utilize sugar, controlling the level of sugar in the blood; it also produces four principal enzymes for digestion: *amylopsin, trypsin, steapsin,* and *rennin.*

8. The *ovaries,* located in the bowl of the pelvis above and on either side of the uterus, produce the female sex hormones *estrogen* and *progesterone.* These account for the more delicate bone structure of the female, the more fully developed breasts, the softer skin and hair, and other feminine characteristics.

THE ENDOCRINE GLANDS

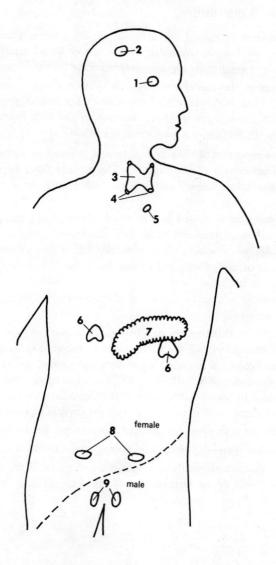

Figure 8

9. The *testes,* located in and below the groin, produce the male sex hormones *testosterone* and *andosterone,* commonly called androgens. These account for the deeper voice of the male, his hairy chest, beard, stronger musculature, and virility.

DISEASES AND DISORDERS

Addison's disease is caused by atrophy of the adrenal glands and is characterized by fatigue, muscular weakness, low blood pressure, nerve impairment, and abnormally pigmented skin on the face and hands.

Adenomas and carcinomas of various glands occur and cover a wide variety of ailments. Tumors or cancers of any one of the endocrine glands will spread rapidly throughout the body because of the wide distribution of the lymphatic fluids from the glands into the blood.

Cretinism is a condition of retarded mental and physical growth, caused by imperfect development of the thyroids. The pulse is slow, metabolism is low, the skin is thickened, and mental and sexual development are retarded.

Cushing's syndrome is caused by overactive adrenal and pituarity glands, resulting in abnormal development in early childhood.

Diabetes insipidus is caused by malfunctioning of the pituitary gland. These is a loss of body fluids and excess thirst, but this disease is not the same as diabetes mellitus.

Diabetes mellitus is due to failure of the pancreas to produce enough insulin to burn up sugar.

Goiter. There are three types: simple, exophthalmic, and toxic. Simple goiter is an enlargement of the thyroid glands due to insufficient iodine. Exophthalmic goiter is the result of excessive thyroxin, and causes rapid heartbeat, shortness of breath, tremors, and protruding eyeballs. Toxic goiter is caused by some malfunction of the thyroids; with this type there are masses of tissue, such as tumors, around the thyroid glands.

Hyperthyroidism is an overproduction of thyroxin by the thyroids.

Hypothyroidism is an insufficient functioning of the thyroids.

Myxedema. Inactive thyroid glands cause a low metabolism, swelling of the face and hands, coarse features, loss of hair, lethargy, and obesity.

TERMINOLOGY

Roots	Terms	Descriptions
aden—	aden/ectomy	removal of any gland
gland	aden/oid/ectomy	removal of the adenoids
adren—	adrenal/ectomy	removal of an adrenal gland
adrenals	adreno/genic	originating in the adrenals
—crine	endo/crine	to secrete within; ductless
secrete	exo/crine	to secrete through a duct
—dema	e/dema	fluid in tissues, swelling
swelling	myx/edema	glandular disease, thyroids
—duct	lympho/cyto/penia	deficiency of lymph cells
opening	lympho/duct	vessel leading from lymph gland
pancreat—	pancreat/itis	inflammation of the pancreas
pancreas	pancreat/olysis	breakdown of the pancreas
parathyroids	para/thyroid/oma	tumor of a parathyroid gland
parathyroids	para/thyro/toxic/osis	toxic disease, parathyroids
physis—	hypo/physis	any process of outgrowth
growth	physi/ology	study of living organisms
pinea—	pineal/oma	tumor of the pineal gland
pineal gland	pinealo/pathy	any disease of pineal gland
pituit—	pituitari/genic	originating in pituitary
pituitary	pituitar/ism	disorder of pituitary action
thyro—	thyro/aden/itis	inflammation of thyroids
thyroid	thyro/toxemia	toxic condition in thyroids

Pronunciations and Accents for Terms

adenogenic	add-en-oh-jen'-ik
adenoma	add-eh-no'-mah
adenectomy	add-en-ek'-to-me
adenotoxicosis	ah-den-oh-tock-si-ko'-sis

(continued)

Pronunciations and Accents for Terms (continued)

adrenal	add-ree'-nal
adrenalectomy	ah-dree-nal-ek'-to-me
adrenogenic	ah-dree-no-jen'-ik
amylase	am'-eh-lace
andosterone	an-dos'-ter-own
carcinoma	kar-si-no'-mah
cirrhosis	seer-oh'-sis
corticotropin	kor'-ti-ko-tro-pin
cretinism	kree'-tin-izm
diuresis	dye-you-ree'-sis
endocrine	en'-do-krin
epinephrine	ep-eh-nef'-rin
estrogen	ess'-tro-jen
exophthalmic	ex-off-thal'-mik
exocrine	ex'-oh-krin
glucagon	gloo'-kah-gon
glycogen	gly'-ko-jen
glycosuria	gly-ko-sure'-ee-uh
histamine	hiss'-tah-meen
hyperinsulinism	high-per-in'-su-lin-izm
hypophysis	high-pof'-eh-sis
insipidus	in-sip'-eh-dus
insulin	in'-sue-lin
lipase	lip'-ace
lymphadenoid	limf-add'-eh-noyd
lymphatolysis	limf-ah-tol'-eh-sis
lymphocytopenia	limf-oh-sit-oh-pee'-ne-uh
lymphoduct	limf'-oh-dukt
lymphostasis	limf-oh-stay'-sis
mellitus	mell-eye'-tus
myxedema	mix-eh-dee'-ma
pancreas	pan'-kree-us
pancreatitis	pan-kree-ah-tye'-tis
parathyroid	pair-ah-thy'-royd
parathyroidoma	pair-ah-thy-royd-oh'-ma
parathyrotoxicosis	pair-ah-thy-ro-tock-si-ko'-sis
parathyroxin	pair-ah-thy-rock'-sin
pineal	pin'-ee-al
pinealoma	pin-ee-ah-lo'-ma

pinealopathy	pin′-ee-al-oh-pathy
pituitary	pit-you′-it-ary
pituitarigenic	pit-you-it-air-eh-jen′-ik
pituitarism	pit-you-′it-air-izm
pituitary	pit-you′-it-ary
progesterone	pro-jes′-ter-own
testes	tes′-teez
testosterone	tes-tos′-ter-own
thymus	thigh′-mus
thyroadenitis	thy-ro-ad-en-eye′-tis
thyrotoxemia	thy-ro-tock-see′-me-uh
trypsin	trip′-sin

REVIEW TEST: THE ENDOCRINE SYSTEM

1. Where are the adrenals located?

2. Where is the thymus located?

3. Where is the pancreas located?

4. Define adenotoxicosis.

5. Define lymphatolysis.

6. Define adenomalacia.

7. Define pancreatitis.

8. Define myxedema.

9. What causes diabetes mellitus?

10. What glands manufacture estrogen?

11. What glands in the male compare to the ovaries in the female?

12. What is known as the "master gland"?

13. Name three types of goiter.

14. Name three diseases of the endocrine system.

15. Differentiate between adenectomy and adrenalectomy.

16. Differentiate between adenitis and adenoiditis.

17. Differentiate between hyperthyroidism and hyperinsulinism.

18. How many parathyroid glands are there?

19. What gland produces insulin?

20. Define lymphocytopenia.

8

THE INTEGUMENTARY SYSTEM

The integumentary system, or the skin, can be thought of as a protective covering, holding in body fluids and keeping out such foreign matter as bacteria. It protects the body from the sun's ultraviolet rays, yet uses sunshine to form vitamin D. It keeps the body cool through perspiration, but also prevents heat loss when the body is exposed to cold. Its millions of nerve endings react to heat and cold, moisture and dryness, pain and pleasure. It is a "wrapping" that can accommodate to changes in shape and size of the body, as it is highly elastic. The skin stretches on a woman during pregnancy, or when one is overweight, yet will go back to its original size after childbirth or weight loss. We can also credit the skin as being a part of sexual attraction, because it identifies each individual by shaping facial and body contours. Fingerprints — the skin's contours over the ends of the fingers and thumbs — are another identifying factor.

The skin rehabilitates itself and heals its wounds. If this were not so, we would all be a mass of scars from scratches, burns, bruises, etc. In animals, the same tissue that produces our epidermis also produces hair, thick hides, nails, claws, beaks, and hoofs. In humans, hair and nails are a part of the integumentary system.

The skin has two layers: the *dermis,* a thick, fibrous mat of tissue, and the *epidermis,* the thin surface coat made up of layers of sheets of cells. The outermost layer is dead tissue, because living cells cannot survive exposure to air and water. If the skin is scratched, tiny scales of dead tissue will flake off. The skin varies in thickness, from the delicate tissue of the inner arm to the coarser skin on the palms of the hands and soles of the feet.

The skin's surface is like a detailed map, marked with ridges, furrows, pores, hair follicles, whorls, and squares. Development of skin begins in the human embryo very early, and at 3 months the fingernails, toenails, and hair follicles begin to form. Males and females have about the same number of hair follicles, but females usually produce smaller and more colorless hairs.

A baby's skin is soft, velvety, clear, and apparently almost hairless. During adolescence, hair follicles, sweat glands, and sebaceous glands become more active. As we grow older, the skin becomes dryer and wrinkled due to years of exposure.

The color of the skin is due to *melanocytes* (color cells), evenly scattered throughout the epidermis. All humans have about the same number of melanocytes, but in dark races, the melanocytes manufacture more melanin. Originally, this adaptation protected the dark races from the tropical sun.

Blood vessels course through the skin all over the body. The sweat glands pour moisture on the skin's surface, and evaporation of this moisture cools the blood circulating through the skin. The skin's blood vessels have tiny sphincter muscles which can shut off the flow of blood, causing blood to flow directly from arteries to veins, acting as a safety valve when blood pressure rises to a dangerous point. A network of nerves in the skin controls both blood vessels and glands. There is also a complex of sensory nerves which respond to tactile and thermal stimuli; without these, we would have much less awareness of the rest of the world.

The hair has some protective functions, too. Hairs inside the nostrils slow incoming air, trap dust particles, keep out insects, and prevent mucus from the nose from dripping. Eyelashes and eyebrows shield the eyes.

The nails of the fingers and toes are composed of layers of horny scales. The nails themselves have no nerves, but the bed of the nail has many nerves and blood vessels, and is sensitive.

The total area of skin on an average human body is about 3000 square inches, or over 20 square feet. This area of protective covering is also a vital body system.

DISEASES AND DISORDERS

Acne. A common skin disorder of adolescence. The sebaceous glands throw off excess oil and a substance called sebum. If the skin is not kept immaculately clean, pustules (infected pimples) form. Hormones along with antibiotics are now being used with some success.

Alopecia. Baldness. There are about 30 different causes of baldness, among them an extremely high fever, injury to the hair follicles, syphilis, nervous diseases, and old age. Baldness is also partly hereditary.

Dermatitis. A blanket term for inflammation of the skin. There are several kinds:

Atopic dermatitis, caused by eczema, nervousness, and scratching, thus causing lesions.

Contact dermatitis, caused by allergy from contact with irritating substances such as dyes, poison ivy, leather, and other products.

Seborrheic dermatitis, an inflammation of the sebaceous glands.

Drug sensitivity. The result of the skin's reaction to drugs to which the patient is allergic or sensitive; basically, the reaction begins in the blood.

Erythema multiforme. A recurrent dermatosis with large red lesions. The causes are many: systemic infection, virus, drugs, allergies, and cancer.

Lupus erythematosus. A grave disease, usually fatal. It is a collagen disease. More than 80% of the victims are women. The disease is rare in the United States. A "butterfly" rash appears on the face, with red areas the shape of butterfly wings on either side of the nose. A variety of other illnesses seem to accompany lupus: pneumonitis, kidney infection, rheumatic fever, anemia, and psychoses. Lupus vulgaris is a tuberculosis of the skin.

Pemphigus. A grave skin disease, nearly always fatal within a few months. Large lesions like blisters appear on the skin and mucous membranes, later become white and flabby as they rupture and spread. The skin sloughs off, and the epidermal cells are destroyed.

Pruritus. A skin irritation characterized by redness, itching, heat, swelling, and tenderness.

Psoriasis. A chronic recurrent dermatitis of unknown cause; the skin becomes red, very dry, and scales off, usually in circular spots.

Scleroderma. Hardened, thickened skin; cause unknown. In the late stages the face becomes masklike, with a pinched nose and difficulty opening the lips. The skin becomes paper-dry, and the fingers stiffen as the skin grows tighter.

Urticaria. Usually called hives. Itching and swelling due to some substance to which the patient is allergic, such as drugs, parasites, plants, foods, or stress and trauma.

TERMINOLOGY

Roots	Terms	Descriptions
cera— wax, waxy	cera/ceous cer/oma	waxlike in appearance a tumor of waxy appearance
cut— *derm—* skin	sub/cut/aneous sclera/derma	beneath the skin hardening of the skin
kerat— scaly	kerato/derma kerato/genesis	scaly skin formation of scaly skin
onych— nail	onych/olysis onycho/phagy	separation of nail from its bed habit of biting the nails
sebum— fat, suet	sebo/lith sebo/rrhea	stone in a sebaceous gland excessive discharge of sebum
squam— plate, scale	squam/ous de/squam/ation	platelike, scaly shedding skin in scales, sheets

Additional Vocabulary

cerumen: ear wax

debridement: removal of dead tissue

hirsutism: abnormal hairiness of the body

keloid: growth of skin due to scar tissue; a raised welt

nummular: coin-shaped, as in a welt

wheal: raised spot on the skin, as in hives

Pronunciations and Accents for Terms

acne	ak'-nee
alopecia	al-oh-pee'-sha
atopic	ay-top'-ik
ceraceous	sear-ay'-shus
ceroma	sear-oh'-mah
cerumen	ser'-you-men
debridement	dee-breed'-ment

dermatitis	der-ma-ty´-tis
dermatosis	der-ma-to´-sis
desquamation	des-kwam-ay´-shun
epidermis	ep-eh-der´-mis
erythema	ear-eh-thee´-ma
erythematosus	ear-eh-thee-ma-to´-sus
follicle	foll´-ik-al
hirsutism	her´-suit-izm
integumentary	in-teg-you-men´-tary
keloid	kee´-loyd
keratoderma	ker-at-oh-der´-ma
lupus	loo´-pus
nummular	num´-you-lar
onycholysis	on-ik-ol´-eh-sis
onychophagy	on-ik-off´-ah-jee
pemphigus	pem´-figus
pneumonitis	new-mo-ny´-tis
pruritus	prew-ry´-tus
psoriasis	soar-eye´-uh-sis
pustule	pus´-tule
scleroderma	skler-oh-der´-ma
sebaceous	see-bay´-shus
sebolith	see´-bo-lith
seborrheic	see-bo-ree´-ik
sebum	see´-bum
squamous	skway´-mus
urticaria	ur-ti-kar´-ee-uh
wheal	wheel

REVIEW TEST: THE INTEGUMENTARY SYSTEM

1. Name three ways the skin serves the body.

2. Name two glands of the skin.

3. Name two layers of the skin.

4. Distinguish between erythema and erythematosus.

5. Distinguish between debridement and desquamation.

6. Locate the mucous membranes of the body.

7. Define subcutaneous.

8. Define scleroderma.

9. Define onychomalacia.

10. Define urticaria.

11. Define alopecia.

12. What gives skin its color?

13. What is a keloid?

14. What is hirsutism?

15. What does squamous mean?

16. Define lupus erythematosus.

17. Name three types of dermatitis.

18. Define pruritus.

19. Define pustule.

20. Describe pemphigus.

REVIEW TEST: CHAPTERS 1–8

Now that you have covered the systems of the body and the terminology applicable to each system, take this review test of the first eight chapters and evaluate yourself on how much you have retained. Define all of the following terms. Some of the terms given here are combinations of components which you have not seen in the text, but if you have memorized the roots, prefixes, and suffixes, you should be able to put the terms together and know their meaining.

Adenotoxicosis

Anterior costodesis

Bilateral nephromegaly

Blepharorrhaphy

Cervical spondylosis

Cholecystonecrosis

Colpoplasty

Craniosclerosis

Cystosarcoma

Dacryolithiasis

Erythrocytosis

Gastroptosis

Hematuria

Heminephrectomy

Hepatomalacia

Hyperinsulinism

Hypoglycemia

Ileogastrostomy

Iliofemoral graft

Laparomyositis

Lumbar spondyloplegia

Lymphocytopenia

Mastectomy

Multiple meningioma

Nephrolithectomy

(continued)

(continued)

Neurofibroma
Onychomalacia
Osteoarthritis
Otorhinopharyngitis
Ovariocyesis
Pancreatolysis
Panleukopenia
Pericardiectomy
Pleuracentesis
Pneumothoracotomy
Posterior cerebrotomy
Postnatal metrorrhagia
Proctoscopy
Sclerodermatitis
Scoliosis
Sialadenitis
Splenomegaly
Stomatitis
Tachypnea
Talipes
Thrombophlebitis
Tracheloma
Tracheorrhexis
Vesiculogram
Viscerotonic

There are 50 terms in this review; grade yourself 2 for each one you have correct. If you have had difficulty with any term, go back and separate it into its components and you should come up with the right answer. If, even then, you cannot define the term, look it up in a medical dictionary. Now you will know where your weaknesses lie in medical terminology, and can concentrate on that portion.

9

PSYCHIATRIC TERMINOLOGY

Psychiatry is so complex that we cannot attempt to do more than become acquainted with the most basic terms. Even these may help us to understand words which have become a part of our everyday language.

Affect and effect. Feelings, emotions, and moods we have *affect* us, in that we become blue, depressed, resentful, and angry, in negative ways, or cheerful, optimistic, and enthusiastic, in positive ways. If we are affected by some incident and suppress this over a period of time, our feelings may reappear in some other form — a nervous habit, a delusion, an obsession, etc.

What *affects* us has an *effect* on us. The effect may be in the form of excessive perspiration, rapid heartbeat or palpitations, weakness, dizziness, nausea, or sleeplessness. It is not abnormal to feel physical effects from things that happen to us. If we did not *react,* we would be subnormal. It is simply a matter of the *degree* to which we let things *affect* us, and how long we suffer from the *effects* of our reactions.

Aggression, or aggressiveness, is a feeling which is expressed in a forceful manner. Aggressiveness describes the person who drives ahead, who fights back when he feels imposed upon, who tries to "run the show," to boss people. This type of person is frequently overcompensating for a feeling of inferiority, but not always.

Passiveness is just the opposite: the person is shy, timid, withdrawn, sits back, says nothing, and hides his feelings. This person usually doesn't have an inferiority complex. In fact, he may feel superior; however, he may be motivated by fear. Both aggressive and passive states, if extreme, may be abnormal, but the aggressive person is likely to be more healthy emotionally, because he does not inhibit his feelings.

Anxiety describes a state of fear, worry, and tension associated with anticipated or imagined danger. It differs from real fear associated with real danger. Anxiety may appear as an emotional or a physical disturbance, in the form of heart palpitation, trembling, labored breathing, tension, etc. In the normal individual, anxiety is felt but is recognized for what it is and soon conquered, whereas in the abnormal type, anxiety persists so long that the person is unable to function in his usual manner.

Conversion is the process by which *emotions* become transferred to *physical* reactions.

Delusion is a false belief that cannot be corrected by logic or reasoning. The delusion cannot be eliminated, in spite of any explanation which would normally be "plain-as-day" evidence. A man may be convinced he has heart trouble, even though a physical examination and an electrocardiogram give ample evidence that his heart is healthy.

Depersonalization is a feeling of unreality about the *self*. The patient subconsciously cannot face reality and feels separated or detached from his familiar self. He feels that he has lost his identity. Such depersonalization is usually brought about by some situation or reaction too painful to face. *Amnesia* (loss of memory) often starts with this feeling.

Depression affects us all at times, for short periods, but the psychiatric term defines a morbid, unrealistic state in which the patient feels his life is useless. There are two types:

Agitated depression: The patient has difficulty in performing the simplest activities, and cannot think clearly. He may stop moving at all and become similar to a catatonic, or he may become frantically active. This state occurs in patients with deep guilt feelings, who are fearful that they or their loved ones will be punished for the act which has caused the guilt feeling. It is this imagined threat of punishment which causes the agitation.

Reactive depression: This is an acute feeling of despondency brought on by some external event such as the loss of a loved one. It differs from the normal disappointment or grief because it is much more pronounced. Sometimes the patient cannot overcome his depression without psychiatric help.

No matter what triggers depression, it is not limited to the mind or emotions; the body is soon affected. Depression has been called "the great masquerader," since it is often the reason behind vague physical complaints for which there seems to be no organic reason. The most common symptoms of depression are headaches, fatigue, loss of appetite, susceptibility to colds, dizziness, gastrointestinal distress, and impotency in men and frigidity in women. No one knows how many old people are simply depressed rather than senile; depression can also cause confusion.

Early recognition of depression is important, for depressed people often don't understand the significance of their feeling and try to pretend it isn't there. When finally they seek medical help, they don't mention depression; some people even deny they feel depressed, thinking their doctor will consider them mentally ill or unbalanced. The doctor who will talk with his patient, explaining the reason for his physical ailments, and encourage him to talk about his worries, can bring much reassurance.

The newest discovery is that people are usually depressed *before* they are ill. Treating the depression helps to treat the illness. Antidepressant drugs — mood elevators — have been of great help in treating arthritis, chronic ulcerative colitis, asthma, and eczema. Victims of Parkinson's disease who were formerly unable to dress themselves were 90% more successful after 3 weeks on antidepressant drugs.

Functional illness is any illness which is not *organic,* but is the result of an emotional disturbance. An organic illness is directly traceable to a physical cause. For example, a rapid heartbeat in organic illness can be caused by damage to the pacemaker of the heart; in a functional illness, the rapid heartbeat is due to fear and has nothing to do with the state of health of the heart itself.

Id: That part of the mind which has to do with instincts; the unconscious.

Subconscious: The deepest part of the mind, the accumulated "racial consciousness" over which we have no control.

Ego: The governing agent of the mind which acts to adjust the savage and the civilized portions of the conscious mind.

Super-ego: The part of the mind which acts as a monitor between the conscious and the unconscious; the *conscience.*

To understand the relationship between these last four terms, visualize a room which is completely dark — blackness impenetrable. Suppose that in one corner of the room a person stands with a flashlight. Where the light shines the brightest is the conscious mind. The blackest corners of the room represent the subconscious mind. The portions of the room which are in partial shadow represent the Id. The person holding the flashlight, who can control its direction of beam, represents the ego and super-ego.

Libido: The energy and drive which comes from our primitive impulses; the motive power behind the sex urge; psychic and emotional energy.

Involutional Psychoses: Involution means turning inward or going backward. Involutional psychoses occur during the years of the female menopause, the male climacteric, or even in later years. This is not the same as *senility* (a kind of feeble-mindedness due to old age), but rather a depression brought on by body changes, hormonal decreases, and a feeling of hopelessness. The emotional troubles that affect a person in his younger years become stronger and deeper in his later years. The better well-balanced emotionally a person is when young, the less likelihood there is for an involutional psychosis when he is old.

Involutional melancholia is a form of involutional psychosis, in which the patient is deeply depressed and melancholy.

Mood swings: The fluctuation between feelings of well-being (euphoria) and depression or feeling badly (malaise). All of us have mood swings, but the neurotic or psychotic personality has mood swings of great intensity.

Neurosis: An emotional disorder not severe enough to be classed as a psychosis. In neurosis only a part of the personality is affected. Symptoms of neuroses may include disturbances in sensory or motor reactions, or developing strange habits, such as being careful not to step on the crack in a sidewalk, or needing to perform daily routines in a definite order or pattern.

Conflict arises when *instinct* urges one to act, but *conscience* warns that the consequences of the act may be bad. A man may be very much attracted to a young woman and want to make love to her, but his conscience tells him that he has a wife and children and cannot do what he wants. This is a conflict between *drives*. Desires and drives that conflict with our conscience may be pushed down into the subconscious. This *repression* may then lead to neurotic behavior because the repressed drive continues to exist on a hidden level and is likely to come out in a distorted, destructive form.

People cope with their conflicts with varying degrees of success: One of the healthiest ways to handle conflict is by *sublimation*. A man with a great deal of aggression may become a battler for a cause; a man who is deeply disappointed not to have had children may be quite paternal toward his employees. Another means is *displacement;* the drive is directed at some other object. A child with a new baby sister may stick pins in her dolls, because subconsciously that's what she'd like to do to the new baby. *Projection* is another outlet for conflict. A disturbed man may shift the blame for his mistakes onto his parents, or to bad luck. A poor workman may claim the boss "has it in for him." Another mechanism is *overcompensation.* The person overcompensates by trying to prove to himself and others that he doesn't have "wicked" drives — the reformed rake becomes a strict moralist; the overly aggressive person becomes a pacifist; the man who doubts his virility becomes a Don Juan.

The main point of this is: don't have guilt feelings if you have drives. We're all born with savage primary urges, feelings from a time when man *was* a savage. Recognize conflict, and accept it. If you can't handle it, see a psychologist, a psychiatrist, or your doctor.

Psyche: The Greek word for soul, now considered to be that part of the mind which adjusts the individual to the needs and the demands of his environment.

Psychoneurosis: The psychoneurotic exhibits the same symptoms as the neurotic except that they are more pronounced. There may be incidents of hysteria, temporary blindness or paralysis, and a compulsive dwelling on fears and anxieties.

Psychosis: A severe mental/emotional illness. There is a definite deviation from the normal pattern of thinking and acting. The personality becomes disorganized, and the world is seen from an unrealistic viewpoint.

Psychology: The science which deals with the study of behavior of mental and emotional processes.

Psychiatry: The science and study of the origin, diagnosis, and treatment of mental and emotional disorders. Psychologists do not have to have an M.D. degree, while psychiatrists must have had four years in medical school, an internship and residency, and in many cases must have been psychoanalyzed themselves.

Psychoanalysis: The long-term process of treating patients by helping them to explore their past emotional experiences, exposing their fears and the facts of their inner life, in order to discover why they have become neurotic or psychotic. The patients are then helped back to a happier way of life by making adjustments to their life situations.

Psychotherapy: A newer method of treating abnormal emotional states by talks with a psychologist or psychiatrist; not as long and extensive a treatment as psychoanalysis, but all that is necessary in most cases. Psychoanalysis may take 3-5 years, whereas psychotherapy is sometimes effective in a matter of weeks or a few months.

Group psychotherapy: The process of talking out one's fears and emotional disturbances in a group of people similarly affected. This method has been most successful because another who has had the same kind of neurosis can often help more than a psychiatrist. This type of therapy now includes concentrated sessions over hours or days, such as T-groups, encounter groups, and sensitivity training.

Psychomotor retardation: A slowing down or abnormal functioning of mental, emotional, and physical reactions; may be due to functional or organic illness, or emotional or physical handicaps.

Psychosomatic: Psyche = mind, *soma* = body; a condition in which the *body* is affected by the *mind*. Anxieties, depression, and neuroses can underlie many of man's illnesses. Modern science has proved that these diseases often have psychosomatic components and may be psychosomatic in origin:

acne	hypertension
angina pectoris	hyperventilation
arthritis	irregular pulse
bronchial asthma	jaundice
circulatory disorders	liver diseases
constipation	low blood sugar
coronary diseases	malnutrition
dermatitis	mucus colitis
diarrhea	overweight
duodenal ulcer	paroxysmal tachycardia
emphysema	peptic ulcer
frequent colds	poor posture
gallbladder diseases	sinusitis
gastrointestinal upset	ulcerative colitis
glandular imbalance	urticaria
headaches	vomiting
heart palpitations	

These diseases are *real*, but they may be brought on by the inseparable interaction between emotions and the body. Psychosomatic medicine is relatively new, but is gaining in importance as science learns more about the relationship between the mind, the emotions, and the body.

Schizophrenia: This mental disease is characterized by almost complete cessation of normal behavior. It is a severe psychosis, marked by a retreat from reality, delusions, hallucinations, and regressive actions. The five major types are:

Catatonic: Almost complete stoppage of body movement. Patients lie or sit in one position for hours or days. The patient may be placed in an awkward position with arm upraised or in a crouch, and will remain so for long periods. Sometimes there are periods of extreme excitement with monotonous repeated movements or sayings.

Hebephrenic: Unpredictable childish behavior, marked disorder in thinking, incoherent baby speech, severe emotional disturbance, wild excitement alternating with deep depression, and vivid hallucinations. This type of schizophrenia usually begins before age 30, and science now believes it may be caused by some chemical imbalance in the brain.

Paranoid: This is the mental patient with convictions of persecution, or a certainty that he has superhuman power. The paranoid is very suspicious, misinterprets every action others make, and believes he is being plotted against. Some paranoids become violent against the people they think are persecuting them. These are also the people who believe themselves to be God, Napoleon, etc. Onset of this type usually occurs between 30 and 40 years of age.

Simple: A chronic form beginning in childhood, also believed to be due to chemical imbalance. The child often refuses to go to school, is antisocial and withdrawn, and has germ phobias about foods, body cleanliness, etc. These patients are unable to cope with life, and unless given early treatment, sometimes become hermits and recluses.

Schizo-affective: An acute form with the combined symptoms of the paranoid and hebephrenic.

Transference: During psychoanalysis or even treatment by a psychologist, at some point the patient, if he follows the average pattern, transfers his fears and guilts to his doctor, making him a scapegoat. Later in the course of treatment he often falls in love with his doctor and feels dependent upon him. As he continues to improve, these feelings diminish and eventually disappear.

Two tests which are used in evaluating emotional balance are the *Rorschach Test* and the *Thematic Apperception Test* (called the T.A.T. among professionals). The Rorschach Test consists of a series of ten ink-blot designs, some black and some in color. The patient is directed to examine each card and tell the person administering the test what he sees in the ink blot. To some people the ink blots resemble animals, birds, and butterflies; to others, the blots look like people, or sex organs. From these responses, a trained evaluator can make an analysis of your personality and emotional balance. The Thematic Apperception Test is a series of photographs which the patient examines one at a time, describing what he thinks might be the story behind the picture. Usually the descriptions are recorded on tape, and then a trained evaluator makes an analysis of the personality and emotional state of the person being tested. The real value of these tests depends almost entirely upon how well trained the analyst is.

Pronunciations and Accents for Terms

amnesia	am-nee'-ze-uh
catatonic	kat-ah-ton'-ik
geriatric	jer-ee-at'-trik
hebephrenic	heb-eh-free'-nik
libido	li-bee'-do
paranoid	pair'-ah-noyd
psychoses	sy-ko'-seez
psychosomatic	sy-ko-so-mat'-ik
Rorschach	Roar'-shak
schizophrenic	skitz-oh-free'-nik
senile	see'-nile
senility	sen-il-'eh-tee
sublimation	sub-lim-ay'-shun

10

PHARMACOLOGY

Since new discoveries are made every year in pharmacology, this listing will not be a final directory. It will cover the basic divisions, so that the student will have a general idea of the areas involved.

ANESTHETICS

These can be divided into four groups: (1.) For inhalation — as before and during surgery; (2.) For injection — intramuscular, intravenous, subcutaneous, spinal; (3.) For oral administration — to be swallowed; (4.) For topical use — on the skin, in the mouth, vagina, and rectum.

For Inhalation

cyclopropane
Fluoromar
Fluothane
halothane
Innovar
Ketaject
methoxyflurane
Penthrane

These are relatively new, volatile gases used for general anesthesia, and require special equipment to administer. Their bases are hydrocarbons and derivatives of ether vapors. They put the patient to sleep rapidly.

nitrous oxide	This is a colorless gas, also called "laughing gas," used for general anesthesia. It is one of the older agents, but still reliable, and used frequently now in combination with one of the newer gases.
chloroform *ether*	These are liquids, the vapors of which are inhaled for anesthesia. Chloroform is dangerous and little used now. Ether is not as commonly used because of its nauseating aftereffects.

For Injection

curare	Distilled from a South American plant and originally used to poison arrow tips, this is a powerful anesthetic and muscle relaxant; it separates the muscle activity from the nerve impulses which activate them. Relaxation can be so deep that respiratory muscles fail to function and breathing can stop. The anesthetist must watch carefully and "bag-breathe" the patient if this happens.
cocaine *Metycaine* *Novocain* *Pontocaine* *Procaine* *tetracaine* *Xylocaine*	All these are amino-benzyl acids and are used in dental surgery for tooth extractions, for regional surgery where general anesthesia is inadvisable or not required, for rectal surgery or inspection, for urethral procedures, and for ophthalmic procedures. They anesthetize a specific, localized area for a short time.
Amytal Sodium *Metycaine* *Pentothal Sodium* *Sarapin* *Seconal*	These are used as sedatives and hypnotics. Amytal, Seconal, and Pentothal are barbiturates. Pentothal Sodium is also called "truth serum." They are slow in their action but long-lasting and relatively safe. Sarapin, a derivative of the pitcher plant, is also a muscle relaxant.

For Oral Administration

Dyclone
Nuporal
Oxaine
Ventussin

These are local anesthetics used for peptic ulcer, and for irritation and inflammation of the mucous membranes of the larynx, bronchi, pharynx, and trachea. They are not curative but relieve the immediate pain.

For Topical (local) Use

Americaine
benzocaine
Novocain
Surfacaine
tetracaine
Unguentine

These and many others with varying brand names are all forms of amino-benzyl (hydrochloric) acid; they are usually ointments and are used for sunburn, burns not too severe to require debridement, hemorrhoids, hives, surface wounds and abrasions, and skin conditions due to allergies. They are also useful in making rectal and vaginal examinations.

ANTIBIOTICS

(See the section on antibiotics preceding Pronunciation Guide.)

chlortetracycline
demethylchlor-
   tetracycline
oxytetracycline
pyrrolidone
   methyltetracycline
tetracycline

This group of antibiotics is cross-resistant, meaning that if one is given and is unsuccessful, others in the group will be unsuccessful. They are broad-spectrum antibiotics derived from *Streptomyces* strains, used for treatment of pneumonia, typhoid fever, urinary-tract infections, meningitis, and streptococcal infections. They may be given orally or by injection.

kanamycin
neomycin
streptomycin
viomycine

These are also derived from *Streptomyces* and are useful in gastrointestinal infections and tuberculosis. They are effective against gram-negative bacteria but are toxic and can cause deafness; they are poorly absorbed from the intestinal tract.

ANTIBIOTICS (continued)

bacitracin
lincomycin
clindamycin
novobiocin
polymyxin
tyrotbrycin
chloramphenicol .

These are useful in staphylococcal infections, are excreted in the urine, and are rapidly absorbed in the intestinal tract. Novobiocin and lincomycin are especially effective for gram-positive bacteria. Polymyxin and bacitracin are toxic to kidneys. These are *not* cross-resistant.

erythromycin
oleandomycin

These three *Streptomyces* derivatives are usually given orally and are effective in most types of respiratory infections. They may be injected also.

ampicillin
cloxacillin
methicillin
nafcillin
oxacillin
penicillin G
penicillin V
phenethicillin

All these are penicillins, derived from the original mold *penicillium*. Most are now synthetics. They are effective in gram-positive and some gram-negative infections. A few people are sensitive to penicillin and can suffer anaphylactic shock, or even death. Some organisms are capable of producing *penicillinase*, an enzyme by-product which neutralizes the antibiotic activity.

SULFONAMIDES

sulfanilamide
sulfadiazine
sulfamerazine
sulfacetamide
sulfasoxizole
sulfapyridine
sulfaguanadine
sulfathiazole
sulfamethizine

These are not classed as antibiotics but are bacteria-inhibiting, and all derive from the original sulfanilamide. They are bacteriostatic rather than bactericidal. While not as sensationally effective as some of the antibiotics, they are not toxic. They were discovered as a component of a red dye, in Germany, in 1934, and until antibiotics came along they were the only life-saving drug for pneumonia and respiratory infections.

ANTIHISTAMINES

Benadryl
  (diphenyldramine)
Chlor-Trimeton
  (chlorpheniramine)
Histadyl
  (methapyrilene)
Ornade
  (chlorpheniramine)
Phenergan
  (promethazine)
Pyribenzamine
  (tripelennamine)
Pyrroxate
  (chlorpheniramine)
Teldrin
  (chlorpheniramine)

These drugs are used to counteract an overproduc-tion of histamine in the body as a result of allergic reaction. Used for hay fever, rhinitis, colds, hives, pruritus, and some forms of allergic dermatitis. They may also contain, in varying quantities, caffein, menthol, ephedrine, and a diuretic drying agent such as ammonium chloride.

ANTISEPTICS
(anti-infectives)

alcohol (70% min.)
Argyrol (liquid)
Butesin Picrate
  (ointment)
carbolic aid
  (liquid, poison)
Furacin
  (nitrofurazine)
gentian violet
  (crystals, poison)
hexachloraphene
  (all forms)
hydrogen peroxide
  (liquid)
iodine (tincture)
Lysol 2%
  (liquid, poison)

Alcohol, carbolic acid, Lysol, and hydrogen peroxide are not only antiseptics when applied to the skin in the right concentration, but are also disinfectants. Argyrol is used chiefly in the eyes and nose. Gentian violet and potassium perman-ganate are used as "soaks" for skin infections and athlete's foot, and as douches. Butesin picrate is used for burns. Furacin, Mercresin, mercuro-chrome, merthiolate, iodine, hydrogen peroxide, Metaphen, and Zephiran are used as general antiseptics in minor cuts, wounds, and abrasions; as sprays or swabs to cleanse areas before surgery; and as genital swabs before childbirth.

(continued)

ANTISEPTICS (continued)

Mercresin (liquid)
Mercurochrome (merbromin)
mercury bichloride
   (liquid, ointment)
Merthiolate (thimerasol)
Metaphen (nitromerasol)
potassium permanganate
   (crystals, poison)
Zephiran
   (benzalkonium chloride)

DRUGS AFFECTING THE HEART AND CIRCULATORY SYSTEM

For Arrhythmias
(abnormal rhythm of heart contractions per minute)

digitalis	This medication is an extract from the foxglove plant; there are at least two dozen brand names, such as Digitoxin, but digitalis is the basis for all. It is used to increase, decrease, or regulate the heartbeat.
quinidine	This is a synthetic sulfate, used to decrease and also regulate the heartbeat.

Vasopressors
(to maintain or elevate blood pressure)

adrenalin
amphetamine
Benzedrine
cyclopentamine
ephedrine
epinephrine
levarterenol
triprolidine

There are about three dozen well-known vaso-pressors, all of which are based on one of these generic products. They are used to maintain normal pressure during anesthesia in surgery or when blood pressure drops due to shock or injury. Vasopressors are also used in smaller amounts when nasal congestion occurs, and an amphetamine — such as Benzedrine — is acceptable as an appetite restricting medication. All have stimulating effects.

Vasodilators
(to dilate or increase the size of blood vessels)

amyl nitrate	Under a trade name such as Serpasil, reserpine is
nitroglycerin	used for hypertension, for toxemias of pregnancy,
rauwolfia	in anxiety-related disorders, and in some psychi-
reserpine	atric disorders. It slows the pulse and has a
	calming effect.

Coagulants
(to prevent hemorrhage)

hesperidin	The purpose of all these is to make it easier for the
prothrombin	blood to clot quickly, thus preventing hemorrhage
thrombin	or stopping it once it has started. Some contain
vitamin K	fibrinogen, a byproduct of blood plasma. All except
	vitamin K must be given intravenously.

Anticoagulants
(to prevent clotting)

Actase	These alter the thickening properties of blood
coumarin	proteins concerned with coagulation and prevent
heparin	clotting. They are used in transfusions and to
warfarin	prevent thrombosis and the formation of embo-
	lisms.

DRUGS AFFECTING THE DIGESTIVE SYSTEM

Antacids

aluminum	Under such brand names as Amphojel, Maalox,
bicarbonate of soda	Gelusil, Mylanta, etc., these drugs act in slightly
calcium salts	different ways to neutralize gastric acids. Pectin,
magnesium salts	being thick and viscous, acts as an absorbent. The
pectin	basic salts of sodium, calcium, magnesium and
sodium salts	aluminum, being alkaline, primarily act by
	neutralizing stomach acid. All are taken orally.

(continued)

DRUGS AFFECTING THE DIGESTIVE SYSTEM (continued)

Digestants

bile salts
enzymes
hydrochloric acid
pepsin

Some diseases and parasites destroy digestive juices. It is necessary to replace these for the person to live. These digestants help to break down the solid states of food and act as catalysts in the extraction of proteins, carbohydrates, and minerals.

Antispasmodics

atropine
bella donna
barbiturates
methscopolamine

These medications calm stomach and intestinal muscles, dry up excess fluids produced during gastrointestinal spasms, and quiet hypermotility, or excessive activity of the gut and stomach.

Emetics

ipecac

mustard and/or
  salt water

Emetics are indicated to induce vomiting, especially when the patient has swallowed certain types of poisons. Poisons which burn should not be vomited if possible since there will be additional burning. These require charcoal, bread, milk, and soothing absorbent materials.

Antinausea Drugs

barbiturates
bella donna
chlorpromazine
Dramamine
Thorazine

Nausea can result from airsickness, seasickness, poison, pregnancy, antibiotics, narcotics, anesthesia, imbalance in the inner ear, and emotional upset. These drugs have a calming effect on the stomach and diaphragm, eliminating the vomiting impulse.

Cathartics and Laxatives

citrate of magnesia

epsom salts

These are cathartics, rather severe in their action. They are saline and tend to dry out the natural intestinal mucosa.

cascara sagrada *castor oil* *phenolphthalein*	These are also cathartics but more severe and irritating to the intestinal mucosa. They are necessary when a thorough cleansing of the intestinal tract is necessary before surgery or X-rays.
agar *milk of magnesia* *mineral oil* *psyllium seed*	These are laxatives, milder in action, useful to "break the habit" of constipation. They are neutralizing in effect, and both agar and psyllium seed add bulk to fecal matter.

DRUGS AFFECTING THE CENTRAL NERVOUS SYSTEM

Depressants

codeine *heroin* *laudanum* *morphine* *opium* *paregoric*	All these drugs have a marked depressing effect on the central nervous system and slow down body processes. Most slow peristalsis, leading to constipation. They also slow down the heartbeat, respiration, and reactions to stimuli. They are of value as analgesics (pain killers) in severe, acute fractures and other traumatic injuries. All are habit forming and addictive.

Psychostimulants or Mood Elevators

deanol acetamidoben- *zoate* *desipramine* *hydrochloride* *imipramine* *hydrochloride* *methylphenidate* *hydrocloride* *pentylenetetrazol* *tranylcypromine*	These drugs are all stimulants to the central nervous system. They are used to relieve the symptoms of depression, and to enhance both mental and physical activities of geriatric patients. Some are also used for children who have minimal brain dysfunction. Their trade names are Benizol, Metrazol, Ritalin, Tofranil, etc.

(continued)

DRUGS AFFECTING THE CENTRAL NERVOUS SYSTEM (continued)

Hypnotics and Sedatives

Amytal
barbiturates
chloral hydrate
Luminal
Nembutal
phenobarbital
Seconal
Thorazine

These drugs are used to quiet nervous states; to treat hyperactivity and hyperemotionalism in mental patients; to eliminate periods of violence; to allow patients under stress to sleep; and to keep postsurgical patients asleep or unaware of their pain. While the brain still receives pain messages, the brain centers which would send back pain alarms are inactivated.

Stimulants

amphetamine
Benzedrine
caffein
Dexedrine

These are the "pep pills" which make people very active, "ready to climb the walls." They are used as dietary medications, as mood elevators, and to activate catatonics or lethargic patients.

Tranquilizers

Compazine
Equanil
Librium
Mellaril
meprobamate
Miltown
Serpasil
Thorazine
Valium

Most tranquilizers are compounds of diazepam or chlorpromazine. While some hypnotics and sedatives are also tranquilizers, none of these tranquilizers are sedatives or hypnotics. These drugs merely calm nervous reactions, give a feeling of well-being, and make it possible for the patient to see his illness in a more objective manner. These drugs have performed miracles in mental hospitals, calming patients who formerly had to be in solitary confinement.

DRUGS AFFECTING THE AUTONOMOUS NERVOUS SYSTEM

Sympathetic Nervous System

adrenalin ephedrine epinephrine Levophed Neo-Synephrine	These drugs are useful in emergency situations; they are heart stimulants and bronchodilators. They relax the smooth muscles of the bronchi, speed up peristalsis, and elevate blood pressure and blood sugar. They are used for asthma, nasal congestion, and some allergies. They can be life-saving.

Anticonvulsants

Dilantin Mesantoin Tridione	These act on epilepsy much as tranquilizers affect mental patients; they calm the nervous centers which bring on attacks, and seem to disconnect brain-centered responses.

DRUGS AFFECTING THE ENDOCRINE GLANDS

acetohexamide: Stimulates the pancreas to produce more insulin.

adrenalin: Inhibits the adrenal glands.

chlorpropamide: Stimulates the pancreas to produce more insulin.

cortisone: Inhibits pituitary secretions and adrenal cortex secretions.

diethylstilbestrol: Estrogen derivative used for prostate diseases.

ergot: Used to control uterine bleeding and uterine contractions.

estrogen: Female sex hormone that replaces ovarian lack of estrogen.

Halotestin: Male sex hormone that replaces deficiencies in male.

insulin: Replaces insulin when pancreatic insulin fails.

iodine: Stimulates the thyroids and prevents goiter.

phenformin: Reinforces inadequate insulin production.

Pituitrin: Replaces an extract from the pituitary gland.

progesterone: Supplementary female sex hormone.

testosterone: Male sex hormone that replaces deficient production.

thyroxin: Replaces thyroid and parathyroid secretions.

tolazamide: Stimulates the pancreas to produce more insulin.

tolbutamide: Stimulates the pancreas to produce more insulin.

VITAMINS AND THEIR USES

Vitamin A: The fat-soluble vitamin, found in carrots, egg yolks, butter, cheese, and yellow vegetables; necessary for good eyesight.

Vitamin B-1: Thiamine; water-soluble; found in liver, meats, malt, and whole grains; this applies to *all* the B-complex vitamins; essential for proper metabolism of carbohydrates.

Vitamin B-2: Riboflavin, a water-soluble vitamin; necessary for proper growth and tissue function.

Vitamin B-6: Pyridoxine, a water-soluble vitamin; important in blood, nervous system and metabolism.

Vitamin B-12: Cyanocobalamin, also water-soluble; vital for prevention of anemia.

Vitamin C: Ascorbic acid, calcium; found in citrus fruits, cabbage, celery, tomatoes, and milk; may help fight off colds; builds bones and teeth.

Vitamin D: Calciferol, a fat-soluble vitamin, called the sunshine vitamin because the body absorbs sunlight to help form it; present in fishliver oils. A deficiency of this vitamin causes osteoporosis and rickets.

Vitamin E: Alpha-tocopherol; fat-soluble; found in fishliver oils, eggs, butter, liver, and wheat germ; function is unknown.

Vitamin F: Fatty acids fall into this group; useful in metabolism of fats.

Vitamin K: Fat-soluble; promotes clotting of blood; found in egg yolks, spinach, and cabbage; now used mostly in synthetic form.

Scientists continue research on vitamins since it is known that there are more vitamins needed and used by the body than are listed here. Good vitamin preparations also include several minerals.

ANTIBIOTICS

Over the centuries scientists have become familiar with and named the hundreds of diseases to which man has fallen victim. For years this list was a random, unclassified collection. Then a Danish physician, Dr. Hans Gram, discovered that some bacteria would take a stain while others would not. He classified all bacteria into two groups: those which took the stain were called gram-positive, and the others gram-negative.

This information had little practical value until 1934, the year penicillin was discovered in England by Dr. Alexander Fleming and developed in the United States. In 1943 Dr. Selman Waksman, in New

Jersey, discovered another antibiotic, streptomycin. Penicillin was found to be most effective against gram-positive bacteria, while streptomycin worked best against gram-negative strains. However, the dividing line was not clearcut, for penicillin worked against some gram–negative bacteria. Streptomycin also developed some side-effects: allergies, sensitivity, and deafness. Bacteriologists speculated that there must be some antibiotic that would inhibit both gram-positive and gram-negative pathogens. Today there are many such antibiotics.

What is an antibiotic? The Greek term means "against life," but in this case bacterial life, not human life. Antibiotics are not rare; they are produced every day in nature by living microorganisms. They're all around us, in the soil, in the air, in rotting vegetation, manure, stagnant pools, and the human gut. In a small dish of dirt the microbe population is greater than the human population of New York City.

Microbes perform many functions: decaying, fermenting, killing each other, and feeding each other. Microbes fight constantly for survival and change continually. They mutate — change shapes and characteristics — in order to live; the changes are permanent, for all the offspring bear the same changes. They thrive on man's waste, as a part of the delicate balance of nature. In this process, some microbes produce substances that kill human disease germs. Consider the millions of years life has existed in some form on this planet. The mind cannot conceive of the number of disease germs in the soil. Why isn't the earth a vast pesthole of dead bodies and disease? — because countless armies of microbes in the soil perform their natural functions, among which is the antibiotic action of killing disease-producing bacteria.

Molds can be used to cure human infection; present-day antibiotics are derived from molds. The Chinese knew this 3000 years ago when they used moldy soybean curd as a cure for infections. The Mayans also used a fungus. Yugoslavian families keep moldy bread in the cellar, and Brazilian Indians have used mold for generations. However, not all antibiotics are suitable for human use: some are powerful enough to cure, and others toxic enough to kill.

Fifty years ago a scientist wrote about an antibiotic he had seen at work, not knowing what he had seen. He was growing bacteria in a test tube; while the bacteria were growing, the liquid in the test tube was cloudy. He left the test tubes uncovered, and a few days later he saw tufts of mold growing on the surface. In a few more days mold covered the entire surface of the liquid; the bacteria in the liquid died and the fluid became clear. At that time it was thought that the bacteria died because the mold cut off the oxygen supply; but the mold had fought a battle for survival against the bacteria, and won — an example of microbial warfare.

Gram-Negative Bacteria

Aerobacter aerogenes
Brucella abortus
Brucella melitensis
Brucella suis
Eberthella typhi
Escherichia coli
Hemophilus influenzae
Hemophilus pertussis
Klebsiella ozogenes
Klebsiella pneumoniae
Malleomyces mallei
Neisseria gonorrheae

Neisseria intracellularis
Pasteurella lepiseptica
Pasteurella pestis
Pasteurella tularensis
Proteus vulgaris
Pseudomonas aeruginosa
Salmonella aertrycke
Salmonella enteritidis
Salmonella paratyphi A.
Salmonella paratyphi B
Salmonella schottmulleri
Salmonella suipestifer
Shigella paradysenteriae
Vibrio comma

Gram-Positive Bacteria

Actinomyces bovis
Bacillus anthracis
Clostridium butyricum
Clostridium perfringens
Clostridium septicum
Clostridium sordelli
Clostridium tetani
Clostridium welchii
Corynebacterium diphtheriae
Diplococcus pneumoniae

Erysipelothrix muriseptica
Myobacterium tuberculosis
Staphylococcus aureus
Staphylococcus fecalis
Staphylococcus hemolyticus
Staphylococcus lactis
Streptococcus fecalis
Streptococcus pyogenes
Streptococcus salivarius
Streptococcus viridans

Definitions of Terms

Bacteria: any round or rod-shaped microorganism (Greek: little rod)
Germ: any pathogenic microorganisms

Microbe: a minute living organism, applied especially to those causing disease, including bacteria and fungi

Microorganism: a microscopic organism, including bacteria, mold, viruses, and yeasts or fungus

Pathogen: any disease-producing microorganism

Pronunciations and Accents For Terms

acetohexamide	ah-see-to-hex'-ah-mide
Actase	ak'-tace
actinomyces	ak-tin-oh-my'-seez
aerobacter	air-ee-oh-bak'-ter
aerogenes	air-oj'-en-eez
aertrycke	air'-trik
aeruginosa	air-oo-gin-oh'-sa
agar	ay'-gar
alpha-tocopherol	al-fa-to-kof'-er-ol
Americaine	ah-mer'-eh-kane
amphetamine	am-fet'-ah-meen
Amphojel	am'-fo-jel
ampicillin	am'-pi-sill-in
amyl nitrate	amill ny'-trate
amytal	am'-eh-tal
analgesic	an-al-jeez'-ik
anesthesia	an-es-thee'-zee-ah
anesthetic	an-es-thet'-ik
anthracis	an'-thra-kis
Argyrol	ar'ji-rol
arrhythmia	ah-rith'-me-ah
atropine	at'-ro-peen
aureus	aw'-re-us
bacillus	ba-sill'-us
bacitracin	bass'-eh-tray-sin
bactericidal	bak-ter-eh-sy'-dal

(continued)

Pronunciations and Accents for Terms (continued)

bacteriostatic	bak-ter-ee-oh-stat'-ik
barbiturate	bar-bit'-you-rate
Benadryl	ben'-ah-drill
benzalkonium	ben-zal-ko'-nee-um
Benzedrine	ben'-zeh-dreen
benzocaine	ben'-zo-kane
bovis	bo'-vis
Butesin Picrate	bew-teh-sin pik'-rate
butyricum	bu-tir'-eh-kum
calciferol	kal-siff'-er-ol
carbamate	kar'-ba-mate
cascara sagrada	kas-kara' sa-grah'-da
chloral hydrate	klor-al hy'-drate
chloramphenicol	klor-am-fen'-eh-kol
chloroform	klor'-oh-form
chlorpheniramine	klor-fen-ear'-ah-meen
chlorpropamide	klor-pro'-pa-mide
chlortetracycline	klor-tet-rah-cy'-kleen
Chlor-Trimeton	klor-try'-meh-ton
citrate	sit'-rate
clostridium	klos-trid'-ee-um
cloxacillin	klok'-sa-sill-in
cocaine	ko-kane'
codeine	ko'-deen
coli	ko'-lee
Compazine	kom'-pa-zeen
Corynebacterium	ko-ri-nee-bak-te'-re-um
coumarin	koo'-mar-in
curare	koo-rah'-rah
cyanocobalamin	sy-an-oh-ko-bal'-ah-min
cyclopentamine	sy-klo-pen'-ta-meen
cyclopropane	sy-klo-pro'-pane
Decadron	dek-'ah-dron
demethylchlortetracycline	de-meth-ill-klor-tet-rah-sy'-kleen
Dexedrine	deks'-ah-dreen
diazepam	dy-ayz'-eh-pam
digitalis	dij-eh-tal'-is
Dilantin	dy-lan'-tin
diphenyldramine	dy-fen-ill-dra'-meen

diphtheriae	dif-theer'-ee-eye
diplococcus	dip-lo-kok'-us
Diuril	dy'-you-ril
Dramamine	dram'-ah-meen
Dyclone	dy'-klone
eberthella	ee-ber-thel'-ah
emetic	ee-met'-ik
enteritidis	en-ter-eh-ty'-dis
ephedrine	ee-fed'-rin
epinephrine	ep-eh-neff'-rin
Equanil	ek'-wa-nil
ergot	err'-got
erysipelothrix	ear-eh-sip'-el-oh-thrix
erythromycin	ee-rith-ro-my'-sin
escherichia	esh-er-ik'-ee-uh
ether	ee'-ther
fecalis	fee'-kal-is
Fluoromar	floo'-ro-mar
Fluothane	floo'-oh-thane
Furacin	few'-rah-sin
Gelusil	jel'-you-sil
gentian	jen'-shun
Halotestin	hay-lo-tes'-tin
halothane	hay'-lo-thane
hemolyticus	hee-mo-lit'-eh-kus
Hemophilus	hee-mof'-el-us
heparin	hep'-ar-in
heroin	her'-oh-in
hesperidin	hes-per'-eh-din
hexachloraphene	hex-ah-klo'-rah-feen
Histadyl	his'-tah-dil
influenzae	in-flew-en'-zye
Innovar	in'-no-var
ipecac	ip'-eh-kak
kanamycin	kan-ah-my'-sin
Ketaject	kee'-tah-jekt
Klebsiella	kleb-see-el'-ah
lactis	lak'-tis
laudanum	law'-da-num

(continued)

Pronunciations and Accents for Terms (continued)

lepiseptica	lep-eh-sep'-tika
levarterenol	lev-ar-ter'-eh-nol
Levophed	lev'-oh-fed
Librium	lib'-ree-um
lincomycin	lin-ko-my'-sin
Luminal	loo'-min-al
Maalox	may'-ah-lox
mallei	mal'-lee-eye
malleomyces	mal-lee-oh-my'-seez
melitensis	mel-eh-ten'-sis
Mellaril	mel'-la-ril
meprobamate	mep-ro-bam'-ate
merbromin	mer-bro'-min
Mercressin	mer-kres'-sin
Merthiolate	mer-thy'-oh-late
Mesantoin	mes-an'-toyn
Metaphen	met'-ah-fen
methapyrilene	meth-ah-py'-ri-lene
methicillin	meth-eh-sill'-in
methoxyflurane	meth-ox-ee-floo'-rane
methscopolamine	meth-sko-pal'-ah-meen
Metycaine	met'-eh-kane
muriseptica	mew-ri-sep'-tika
Mycobacterium	my-ko-bak-teer'-ee-um
Mylanta	my-lan'-ta
nafcillin	naf'-sil-in
Neisseria	ne-ser'-ee-uh
Nembutal	nem'-bu-tal
neomycin	nee-oh-my'-sin
Neo-Synephrine	neo-si-nef'-rin
nitromerasol	ny-tro-mer'-ah-sol
nitrous oxide	ny-trus ox'-ide
novobiocin	no-vo-bi'-oh-sin
Novocain	no'-vo-kane
Nuparal	nu'-par-al
ozogenes	oh-zoj'-en-eez
paradysenteriae	pair-ah-dis-en-ter'-ee-eye
paratyphi	pair-ah-ty'-fee

paregoric	pair-eh-gor′-ik
Pasteurella	pas-tew-rel′-lah
pectin	pek′-tin
penicillin	pen-eh-sill′-in
penicillinase	pen-eh-sill′-eh-nace
Penthrane	pen′-thrane
Pentothal	pen′-to-thal
perfringens	per-frin′-jenz
permanganate	per-mang′-ah-nate
pertussis	per-tus′-sis
Phenergan	fen′-er-gan
phenethicillin	feen-eth′-eh-sill-in
phenformin	fen-for′-min
phenobarbital	fee-no-bar′-bi-tal
phenolphthalein	fee-nol-thay′-leen
pituitrin	pi-tu′-eh-trin
polymyxin	polly-mix′-in
Pontocaine	pon′-to-kane
Procaine	pro′-kane
promethazine	pro-meth′-ah-zeen
Proteus	pro′-tee-us
prothrombin	pro-throm′-bin
Pseudomonas	su-do-mo′-nus
psyllium	sil′-lee-um
pyogenes	py-oj′-eh-neez
Pyribenzamine	peer-eh-ben′-za-meen
pyridoxine	peer-eh-dox′-een
pyrrolidone	peer-rol′-eh-done
Pyrroxate	py-rock′-sate
quinidine	kwin′-eh-deen
rauwolfia	raw-wol′-fee-uh
reserpine	res′-er-peen
riboflavin	ry′-bo-flay-vin
salivarius	sal-eh-var′-ee-us
Salmonella	sal-mo-nell′-ah
Sarapin	sair′-ah-pin
schottmulleri	shot′-mull-er-ee
Seconal	sek′-oh-nal
septicum	sep′-ti-kum

(continued)

Pronunciations and Accents for Terms (continued)

Serpasil	ser'-pa-sil
Shigella	shi-gel'-lah
sordelli	sor-dell'-ee
spiramycin	spy-rah-my'-sin
staphylococcus	staf-eh-lo-kok'-us
stilbestrol	stil-bes'-trol
streptococcus	strep-to-kok'-us
streptomycin	strep-to-my'-sin
suipestifer	swee-pes'-ti-fer
suis	swees
sulfacetamide	sul-fa-see'-ta-mide
sulfadiazine	sul-fa-dy'-ah-zeen
sulfaguanadine	sul-fa-gwah'-na-deen
sulfamerazine	sul-fa-mer'-ah-zeen
sulfamethizine	sul-fa-meth'-eh-zeen
sulfanilamide	sul-fa-nil'-ah-mide
sulfapyridine	sul-fa-py'-ri-deen
sulfasoxizole	sul-fa-sox'-eh-zole
sulfathiazole	sul-fa-thy'-ah-zole
Surfacaine	sur'-fo-kane
Teldrin	tel'-drin
tetani	tet'-an-ee
tetracaine	tet'-ra-kane
thiamine	thy'-ah-meen
thimerosal	thy-mer'-ah-sol
Thorazine	tho'-ra-zeen
tolazamide	toll-ay'-za-mide
tolbutamide	toll-bu'-ta-mide
tripelennamine	try-pel-en'-ah-meen
tripolidine	try-poll'-eh-deen
tularensis	tu-lah-ren'-sis
typhi	ty'-fee
tyrothrycin	ty-ro-thry'-sin
Unguentine	ung'-gwen-teen
Valium	val'-ee-um
Ventussin	ven-tuss'-in
Vibrio	vib'-ree-oh
viridans	veer'-eh-danz
vulgaris	vul-gar'-is

warfarin	war'-fair-in
welchii	wel'-chee-eye
Xylocaine	zy'-lo-kane
Zephiran	zef'-ear-an

11

THE CASE HISTORY AND PHYSICAL EXAMINATION QUESTIONNAIRE

Before the physician performs his physical examination of a patient, either he or his nurse should take the patient's case history. As a guide for these two procedures, a typical case history and physical examination questionnaire follows below. (The patient is an imaginary one.)

Case History

Date   *Aug. 1, 1973*   Name   *Marilyn Barre*

Referring physician   *H. J. Rand, MD*

Insurance   *Blue Cross*

Patient's address   *14375 Cactus Rd., Greensville*

Telephone   *740-3811*   Blood type   *0+*

Date of birth   *Mar. 29, 1939*   Race *Caucasian*

Place of birth   *San Francisco, Calif.*

(continued)

Case History (continued)

Marital status   *Married*   Spouse   *John Barre*

Children   *3*   Occupation   *Accountant*

Employer   *Wilby and Son*

Name and address of family physician or previous doctor   *H. J. Rand,*
   Mills Court, Greensville

When did you last consult a physician?   *one year ago*

For what purpose?   *headaches, nausea*

Have you ever had chest X-rays or other X-rays?   *yes*

When and for what purpose?   *previous surgery*

Have you ever had an electrocardiogram?   *yes*

When and for what purpose?   *general physical examination*

   Childhood diseases: Measles, mumps, whooping cough, chicken pox — no aftereffects. No rheumatic fever, scarlet fever, or diphtheria.

   Immunizations: Smallpox, Salk vaccine, diphtheria, tetanus, TB, typhoid.

   Major illnesses: Had lobar pneumonia about 6 years ago; good recovery; no recurrence.

   Accidents and injuries: Fracture of right anterior tibia 15 years ago.

   Surgery: T & A, age 8; appendectomy, age 20; 3 children, no abnormalities.

   Allergies: Penicillin, citrus fruits.

   Family history: Mother living and well, age 62. Father living and well, some arthritis, age 68. One brother living and well, age 38. Two sisters living and well, ages 32 and 36. No family history of tuberculosis, carcinoma, epilepsy, or mental diseases. One paternal aunt is a diabetic.

   Personal history: Patient is married, has 3 children living and well. Has been married 15 years, rates marital relations as "just average." Regards herself as conscientious and hard working. Keeps house for her family and works as an accountant. Smokes about a pack a day of cigarettes. Considers herself a social drinker. Family has some large debts and patient is concerned about this. Children: son, age 12, full-term normal birth; daughter, age 10, full-term breeched birth; daughter, age 6, full-term normal birth.

Sociopsychological outlook: Patient admits she worries too much and probably doesn't get sufficient sleep. Feels the family social life is too restricted, partly due to her working and using evenings for housework. Feels shaky and nervous at times, has difficulty sleeping. Has a poor appetite, occasional diarrhea. Menstrual periods regular and normal, no excessive flow.

Current medications: Family doctor prescribed Librium several weeks ago. Occasionally takes milk of magnesia, and aspirin daily.

PHYSICAL EXAMINATION

Chief complaint: This 34-year-old white female was in good health until about a month ago when she began to have discomfort in the epigastric region, with nausea. She states her discomfort is worse an hour or two after eating and is somewhat relieved by food. Has had some relief from a mild, bland diet and antacids. Pain seems fairly well localized, does not radiate to posterior or costal areas. For the past week she has had a feeling of fatigue and nervousness. No melena or bright red blood in urine or stools. No history of jaundice or gallbladder disease, no history of similar difficulties other than mild indigestion. She has lost 7 pounds in the past two weeks, which she attributes to loss of appetite.

Patient has been under some stress at home and at work recently. An illness in her family has caused some worry. No chills, fever, or night sweats.

Temperature: 98.6   **Pulse:** 88   **Respiration:** 22+
Height: 5'4"   **Weight:** 108   **Blood pressure:** 110/80

Head: Scalp healthy, hair fine and dry. Frequent headaches, probably from tension.

Eyes: Patient has worn glasses for 5 years. No recent vision changes; no blurring, double vision, or pain in or back of eyes. No exudates. Eyes react normally to light. No photosensitivity.

Ears: No deafness, discharge, or vertigo. Drums and ear canals normal.

Case History (continued)

Nose, throat, and mouth: No nosebleeds. Frequent colds during winter months, occasional sinus congestion. Mucous membranes normal. Teeth in good repair.

Neck: Supple, good carotid pulsations bilaterally. Thyroids not palpable. No adenopathy. No venous distention. Slight tension in cervical spine.

Chest: Breath sounds slightly diminished. Some hyperresonance to percussion. No rales. Lungs clear on auscultation. No chest pain or chronic cough.

Heart: No murmurs, normal sinus rhythm. No palpitations. Pulse within normal range, respiration at upper limits of normal.

Gastrointestinal: No distention of abdomen. Well-healed lower right quadrant scar. Tenderness to epigastrum on palpation. No severe digestive difficulties. Tendency toward diarrhea, some flatulence.

Kidneys: Not palpable.

Spleen: Not palpable.

Liver: Palpable but not enlarged. No A-P tenderness.

Genitalia: No masses; vagina and labia normal. Pelvic examination reveals slight tear in cervix; uterine cautery indicated. Ovaries palpable and normal, no cysts or fibroids.

Urinary: No frequency of urination, no pain, no blood in urine. No history of enuresis, dysuria, or nocturia. Bladder not palpable. Urinalysis within normal range.

Rectal: Sigmoidoscopy reveals no polyps. Sphincter tone good, no melena or fresh blood in stools. No rectal masses, slight hemorrhoids.

Bones and joints: No bursitis or joint tenderness. No swelling, good range of motion of extremities, good flexion and extension. No swelling or rheumatic tendencies. Joints normal, no enlargement.

Neurology: Tendon reflexes brisk and symmetrical. Negative Babinski. No history of fainting, convulsions, or coma.

Menstrual history: Menses began at age 13. Dysmenorrhea which subsided after birth of first child. Some low back pain during period. No edema.

Impression: Upper abdominal pain with nausea. Emotional stress.

Program: Patient hospitalized for G-I workup and diagnostic study. Management with Pamine and Librium 25 mg q.i.d. Bland ulcer-type diet. Antacids between meals and at bedtime. A-P and lateral X-rays, barium enema and fluoroscopic studies ordered. F.B.S., BUN, BMR, CBC, ESR. Gallbladder and liver function tests ordered.

NOTE TO THE STUDENT: Now that you have read through the case history and physical examination questionnaire, go back and read it again, underscoring each medical term you find. If you cannot give the layman's meaning for the term, look it up and be sure you understand it.

On some physicians' examinations, there will appear at the end of the dictation or tape, or on a sheet of paper, the following symbols or orders:

Bilirubin ( )	* Prothrombin c.t. ( )
Cephalin flocculation ( )	Electrocardiogram ( )
Serum iron ( )	Acetone ( )
Urinalysis ( )	Serum total protein ( )
BMR ( )	Creatinine ( )
CBC ( )	ESR ( )
Papanicolaou ( )	Liver function ( )
Albumin ( )	Uric acid ( )
Calcium ( )	† BSP ( )
BUN ( )	EEG ( )

* Prothrombin c.t.: Abbreviation for prothrombin consumption test; a test to determine residual serum prothrombin after blood coagulation.
† BSP: abbreviation for bromsulphalein test.

These are all tests, one or more of which he may want the hospital to perform. If you are working for a physician or are going to be working for one, it is wise to memorize these.

Notice also that the physician in the sample Physical Examination did *not* give a diagnosis; he merely gave an "impression." His diagnosis would not be given until the patient had all the tests ordered and he had an opportunity to observe her for a few days.

This review should give you specific evidence of where your weakness lies in the study of the preceding text. Mark one for each question you answer correctly. No answer sheet is given; you should look at the body system related to the term to confirm your answers.

Give the proper term for the description:

1. Cancer of the gallbladder

2. Hardening of liver tissue

3. Painful or difficult swallowing

4. Suture of any muscle

5. Abnormally enlarged head

6. Excessive sugar in the blood

7. Inflammation of veins with clots

8. Hernia of the bladder

9. Inflammation of abdominal muscles

10. Stoppage of blood flow

11. Breakdown of kidney tissue

12. Plastic surgery on the lip

13. Inflammation of cheeks and gums

14. Surgical incision into chest

15. Blood in the urine

16. Surgical removal of half the stomach

17. Pain in the breast

18. Removal of kidney stones

19. Surgical puncture of the skull

20. Surgical removal of an ovarian cyst

21. Abnormally enlarged liver

22. Dropping downward of the stomach

23. Softening of the bones

24. Plastic surgery on both ears

25. Surgical removal of a hip bone

26. Cancer of the bone marrow

27. More or less permanent opening in colon

28. Deficiency of lymph cells

29. Surgical puncture of a lung

30. Paralysis of the bladder

31. Hemorrhage from the nose

32. Painful or difficult speaking

33. Removal of half a kidney

34. Inflammation of the gallbladder

35. Softening of spine

36. Tumor involving muscle & cartilage

37. Excessive fat cells in blood

38. Hardening of the arteries

39. Excessive sugar in the urine

40. Softening of fingernails

41. Rupture of a blood vessel or vein

42. Inflammation of many nerves

43. High blood pressure

44. Fibrous ovarian tumor

45. Inflammation of a heart valve

46. Incision into the brain

47. Surgical fixation of a joint

48. Paralysis of the spine

49. Surgical fixation of a kidney

50. Suture of an eyelid

Define these terms:

51. Dacryorrhea

52. Tachycardia

53. Pericardiectomy

54. Hypoglycemia

55. Urostasis

56. Stomatitis

57. Myeloma

58. Metrorrhagia

59. Laparomyositis

60. Osteogenic

61. Hysteropexy

62. Trachelosarcoma

63. Sialadenitis

64. Pneumonolysis

65. Urethritis

66. Mammectomy

67. Hepatomalacia

68. Tracheotomy

69. Proctoscopy

70. Leukocytosis

71. Dactyloplegia

72. Psoriasis

73. Dacryadenitis

74. Blepharorrhaphy

75. Gastroenterostomy

76. Cholecystectomy

77. Hypothyroidism

78. Diverticulitis

79. Osteomyelitis

80. Bronchiectasis

81. Rhinoplasty

82. Otorhinopharyngitis

83. Pyonephritis

84. Myelocytopenia

85. Dysuria

86. Adenotoxicosis

87. Lymphocytopenia

88. Amenorrhea

89. Myocarditis

90. Pneumothoracic

91. Tracheorrhexis

92. Ileonecrosis

93. Odontalgia

94. Bradycardia

95. Iridocele

96. Cystoscopy

97. Dysmenorrhea

98. Enterocolitis

99. Adrenalectomy

100. Desquamation

FINAL EXAMINATION

Multiple choice: circle the correct term

1. Paralysis of the bladder:

   cytoplagia   nephrostasis   cystoplegia   uroplegia

2. Hemorrhage from the kidney:

   pyelorrhexis   hepatorrhagia   nephrorrhagia   nephrorrhea

3. Softening of the spine:

   osteomalacia   spondylomalacia   spondylolysis   arthromalacia

4. Blood in the urine:

   hematuria   dysuria   hyperglycemia   uremia

5. Abnormally enlarged liver:

   nephromegaly   hepatomegaly   cystomegaly   adrenomegaly

Matching terms: place the correct letter in the open space

6. ( ) Inflammation of abdominal muscles   A. Bradycardia

7. ( ) Abnormally slow heartbeat   B. Cholecystectomy

8. ( ) Surgical fixation of the spleen   C. Splenopexy

9. ( ) Tumor in the mouth   D. Laparomyositis

10. ( ) Surgical removal of gallstones   E. Stomatoma

Define each term in as few words as possible:

11. Cardiovalvulitis

12. Craniotomy

13. Gastroptosis

14. Sialadenitis

15. Lymphocytopenia

Give the correct term for the description:

16. More or less permanent opening in colon

17. Breakdown of pancreatic tissue

18. Hardening of the skin

19. Constant flow of tears

20. Excess fluid in fingers & toes

LANDMARKS IN THE HISTORY OF MEDICINE

Radioactive isotopes and atomic instruments have made it possible to know that the evolution of man began about a million years ago. The anthropoids began 600,000 years ago. Neanderthal man lived 200,000 years ago, and that's when the first knowledge of medicine began. Menaced daily by falling boulders and wild beasts, man learned to do something about pain. Wounds were licked, bleeding was stopped with a pack of mud, painful joints were baked before a fire; fevered bodies were cooled by diving into icy streams. Broken bones were wrapped in leaves, held rigid by twigs – the first bandages and splints.

After living for centuries in caves, the end of the Mesolithic age came 12,000 years ago. Man began living in tribes, building log and thatch huts for shelter. About 7000 B.C. man exchanged a hunter's life for agriculture and began using remedies of water, steam, and herbs. Now that men were living closer together and keeping dogs and other warm-blooded animals, he began to be the victim of bacteria which had formerly lived only on animals. He believed illness was caused by evil spirits, and the medicine man was called upon for counter-magic. The medicine man's therapeutic armamentarium consisted of shells, stones, animal bones, roots, bark, seeds, herbs, and fermented sap. Wounds were stitched with animal sinews and fastened with thorns. Skulls were trephined and the rondelle – the top of the skull – removed to relieve headaches and let out evil spirits. The miracle is that men survived this primitive surgery.

By 3000 B.C. the Egyptian civilization brought medicine a long way forward. The apothecaries (then doctors, now pharmacists) had collections of about 800 prescriptions. Most were made of herbs, but they worked relatively well.

In 400 B.C. Aristotle, the Greek philosopher and physician, and his pupil Dioscorides collected and described all the medications known at that time. Their book, *The Doctrine of Signatures,* was used throughout the world until almost the beginning of the twentieth century. Hippocrates began the practice of "humerus" medicine about the same time. He believed all diseases were due to humors, or body fluids.

In 300 B.C. the practice of medicine was centered in monasteries. The ancient Egyptian and Greek books were translated into Latin for the monastery libraries; the teaching of medicine as a science began with the Benedictine monks.

About 54 A.D. the Arabs began their contribution to medicine. They made the separation between physicians and pharmacists by establishing the first pharmacies to serve physicians.

In 700 A.D. in Salerno, south of Naples, four physicians began a school. One physician was Greek, one Italian, one an Arab, and one a Jew, thus representing the four great cultures of that time. Other doctors, teachers, and translators made up the faculty. Nuns taught about women's diseases and midwifery. This first medical school required three years of "logic," five years of medicine, and one year of practice to earn a certificate — very much like our present four years of college, four years of medical school, and a year in internship. We now require a residency as well.

By 1200 A.D. this school and others founded by monasteries taught anatomy, physiology, pathology, therapeutics, surgical procedures, diets, and health hygiene. Diets recommended prunes dipped in wine for breakfast, chopped onions for growing hair, garlic for menstrual cramps. It was advised that bathing was harmful. In this century clinical case histories were started and medical literature began to collect.

In 1315 Mondion Luzzi, an Italian, initiated the systematic dissection of cadavers to teach anatomy. In 1360 a French physician, Guy de Chauliac, developed the treatment of fractures with splints, slings, and traction. Before this time, barbers were about the only surgeons; the red-and-white striped barber pole originated to indicate to passers-by where the barber-surgeon was located.

In the fourteenth century Oxford University was founded. Here the Dominican Friar Roger Bacon developed the microscope and eye glasses. Oxford's School of Medicine became famous for its comprehensive courses.

Late in the fourteenth century two terrible plagues swept through Europe — the Black Death, or bubonic plague, and leprosy. People either died of the plague in three days or the disease lasted about two months, with high fever, bloody sputum, abscesses, and carbuncles or boils. The Black Death killed between half and three-quarters of the people of Europe. Leprosy came from the Near East to Sicily and spread throughout Europe before it was checked by the founding of separate leper colonies. These two diseases brought about a revolution in sanitation and medicine. Hot baths were the vogue. Physicians prescribed enemas, purges, emetics — every cleansing procedure possible. Streets were swept, and bakeries, meat and fish markets, and vegetable stalls were inspected for sanitary conditions.

The Renaissance began in 1400, and by the time Columbus had discovered America a new age was well under way. Now medicine began to be truly a science instead of a collection of remedies. King James of England granted the first charter for a guild of apothecaries. In 1640 John Winthrop, Governor of Massachusetts Bay Colony, gave recognition to physicians in America. In 1751 Benjamin Franklin helped to establish the first American hospital at Philadelphia. John Morgan, the pharmacist at this hospital, introduced the writing of prescriptions and defended the separate and independent practice of pharmacy.

In 1780 Carl Scheele of Sweden discovered oxygen, tungsten, nitroglycerin, and many other compounds. He paved the way for two important events: Friedrich Serturner, a German scientist, found the narcotic principle of opium and discovered the importance of alkaloids, and Pelletier, a young French doctor, discovered the medicinal qualities of strychnine and quinine.

In 1846 Guy Morton developed anesthesia. In 1886 Limousin, a pharmacist, devised the medicine dropper, the hypodermic syringe, the gelatin capsule, an apparatus to administer oxygen, and a glass ampoule which could be sealed and sterilized for injections. In 1895 Louis Pasteur founded the science of microbiology and developed the process now called pasteurization. In 1910 Dr. John Murphy produced the first scalpel with disposable blades. In 1912 Joseph Lister discovered the powerful bactericidal qualities of antiseptics. Pasteur was the first to discover antibiotic action in 1877, but it wasn't until Dr. Alexander Fleming discovered penicillin in 1934 that antibiotics were fully understood.

While Fleming was working on penicillin, a scientist named Danagk, in a chemical plant in Germany, found that a red dye called protosil killed pneumococci. He experimented until he found that the color molecule of the dye was attached to a molecule of sulfonamide. Thus began the sulfanilamides, which until penicillin was perfected, were the only life-saving drugs for pneumonia and strep throat infections.

In 1943, at Rutgers University, Dr. Selman Waksman discovered streptomycin in one of hundreds of soil samples, and we emerged into the field of broad-spectrum antibiotics.

Mention must also be made of the father of psychiatry, Dr. Sigmund Freud, who began his work in Vienna in 1876, and of his fellow psychiatrists Alfred Adler (1900) and Carl Jung (1905), and the many other profound psychiatrists of the twentieth century.

More progress has been made in medical science in the first 70 years of this century than in the entire previous history of man — and the door to knowledge has hardly begun to open.

RECOMMENDED READING LIST

This is not a bibliography but a list of books, both fiction and nonfiction, concerning various facets of the medical world. A layman can learn much about medical practice from these books.

Note that The Readers' Digest Condensed Version numbers have been included here for the student pressed for time, because this version shortens reading time while still providing the main points of the book.

Baker P: *The Antibodies.* New York, GP Putman's Sons, 1969; paperback by Berkley Medallion Books, 1971. A novel about the fight to control organ rejection in transplants by trying to learn more about the immunosuppressive processes of the body.

Barnard C: *One Life.* New York, Macmillan Company, 1969; Readers' Digest Condensed Version, Volume 3, 1970. The true story of the life of a great pioneer in heart transplants.

Curie E: *Madame Curie.* New York, Doubleday & Company, 1937; Readers' Digest Condensed Version, Volume 2, 1961. The true story of the life of Madame Curie and the discovery of radium.

deKruif P: *Microbe Hunters.* New York, Harcourt Brace & World, 1962; paperback by Pocket Books, Inc. The history of several microbiologists and their searches.

"Doctor X": *Intern.* New York, Harper & Row, 1965; Readers' Digest Condensed Version Volume 3, 1965. The story of one doctor's internship and all it involved. (The writer remains anonymous.)

Fromm E: *The Art of Loving.* New York, Harper & Row, 1956; paperback by Pocket Books, Inc., 1963. Not a sex book but one on the philosophy of love as it applies to psychological health.

Fromme A: *Our Troubled Selves*. New York, Farrar Straus & Giroux, 1967. A very helpful book about understanding ourselves emotionally and how to stay emotionally healthy.

Gordon N: *The Death Committee*. New York, McGraw-Hill Book Company, 1969; Readers' Digest Condensed Version, Volume 3, 1969. A book about a group of doctors, their rounds, their problems, and information on postmortems.

Hailey A: *The Final Diagnosis*. New York, Doubleday & Company, 1959; Readers' Digest Condensed Version, Volume 2, 1960. A novel about doctors, thoroughly researched by a writer significant in his field.

Heinz WC: *The Surgeon*. New York, Doubleday & Company, 1963; Readers' Digest Condensed Version, Volume 2, 1963. A novel about two surgeons, one on the edge of retirement, one just starting out – their cases, problems, and disagreements.

Hodgins E: *Episode*. New York, Atheneum Books, 1963; Readers' Digest Condensed Version, Volume 4, 1964. One man's true story of a stroke he suffered, its consequences, and his rehabilitation.

Mayo CW: *Mayo*. New York, Doubleday & Company, 1968; Readers' Digest Condensed Version, Volume 2, 1969. The story of the famous Mayo brothers and the Mayo Clinic.

Miller BF: *The Modern Medical Encyclopedia*. New York, Golden Press, 1965, Volumes I-XII. This set of medical books written specifically for the layman can be a valuable reference set for a person employed in a medical field.

Powell J: *Why Am I Afraid to Tell You Who I Am?* Argus Books, Chicago, 1969. Philosophy and psychology – perceptive.

Redlich F, Bingham J: *The Inside Story*. New York, Vintage Books, 1953. An immensely entertaining and provocative book about why we behave as we do, written by a psychiatrist and a layman.

Schutz WC: *Joy*. New York, Grove Press, 1967. The story of T-groups, encounter groups, and what they can do for the individual.

Shepard M, Lee M: *Marathon 16*. New York, George Putman's Sons, 1970; paperback by Pocket Books, Inc., 1971. Another story of encounter groups, and how the members react and interact.

Thigpen CA, Cleckley HM: *The Three Faces of Eve*. New York, McGraw Hill Book Company, 1957; Readers' Digest Condensed Version, Volume 3, 1957. The fascinating true story of a woman with three distinct personalities, and how she was cured.

Thompson M: *Not As A Stranger*. New York, Charles Scribner's Sons, 1954; Readers' Digest Condensed Version, Volume 2, 1954. The story of a man from premed-school days through almost all the rest of his life.

Thorwald J: *The Century of the Surgeon*. New York, Pantheon Books, 1957; Readers' Digest Condensed Version, Volume 4, 1957. The fascinating history of surgery.

Thorwald J: *The Triumph of Surgery*. New York, Pantheon Books, 1960; Readers' Digest Condensed Version, Volume 1, 1960. Another absorbing book about surgery by the same excellent author.

Woodham-Smith C: *Florence Nightingale*. New York, McGraw-Hill Book Company, 1951; Readers' Digest Condensed Version, Volume 3, 1963. The authentic life story of the first and famous nurse.

Young A: *The Town and Doctor Moore*. New York, Simon & Schuster, 1966; Readers' Digest Condensed Version, Volume 1, 1967. The life story of an old-fashioned "family doctor" or general practitioner and what he accomplished.

74 75 76 77 78 10 9 8 7 6 5 4 3 2 1